THE COMPLETE FAMILY GUIDE TO SURVIVING PROSTATE CANCER: A JOURNEY OF HOPE AND HEALING

Treatments Book For Recovery

first edition

By
Arnold D. Rosenthal, M.D., PH.D.,
Dr Ben T. Murray & Mandy L.Carson

COPYRIGHT

Table of Contents

INTRODUCTION

5

You might be reading this book because you have been diagnosed with prostate cancer, or perhaps your Prostate-Specific Antigen (PSA) levels have been rising, making you anxious that tumor or malignancy may be imminent. Alternatively, you could be reading this for a friend or family member, examining the available treatment choices and pondering the next course of action.

Regardless of what led you to this book, "The Complete Family Guide to Surviving Prostate Cancer" you are warmly received and welcome

This book bears the collective wisdom of three individuals who have dedicated their lives to understanding and combating prostate cancer. Yet, amidst the esteemed

6

voices of experts, there lies the voice of personal experience—my own.

A Family's Journey with Prostate Cancer: The Arnold Story

In 1985, my grandfather, Fred Arnold, was diagnosed with stage 4 prostate cancer at the age of 65. At that time, the symptoms were severe and unmistakable. He experienced intense pain in his bones, frequent and urgent urination, difficulty starting and stopping the urine stream, blood in his urine, and extreme fatigue. These symptoms indicated that the cancer had spread beyond the prostate, affecting other parts of his body.

During the mid-1980s, knowledge about prostate cancer was limited, and specialized treatments were not as advanced or readily available as they are today. Healthcare providers struggled to understand the disease, often resorting to experimental or poorly understood treatments. My grandfather was subjected to a series of harsh and unproven therapies. He underwent radical prostatectomy, which was a risky and invasive surgery at the time. The procedure was followed by early forms of radiation therapy that were not precisely targeted, causing significant collateral damage to surrounding healthy tissues.

In addition to surgery and radiation, my grandfather was given hormone therapy, which involved the use of medications to drastically reduce testosterone levels. These treatments had severe side effects, including hot flashes, loss of libido, and significant bone thinning. Despite these aggressive measures, the cancer continued to spread, and my grandfather's health deteriorated rapidly.

The lack of expertise and appropriate treatment options meant that Fred Arnold endured a great deal of suffering. The healthcare system at the time was not equipped to handle such advanced cases of prostate cancer, leading to treatments that were often more harmful than beneficial. My grandfather spent his final months in considerable pain, and the family watched helplessly as he succumbed to the disease. He passed away within a year of his diagnosis, a tragic outcome that reflected the limited medical knowledge and resources available at the time.

This experience had a profound impact on our family. My father, Douglas Arnold, was determined to stay informed about prostate cancer, especially as he approached the age when the risk increased. When he turned 50, he started regular screenings, including prostate-specific antigen (PSA) tests and digital rectal exams (DREs), to catch any early signs of the disease.

In 2010, at the age of 60, my father was diagnosed with prostate cancer. Unlike his own father, he was fortunate to benefit from significant advancements in medical science. The cancer was detected early, thanks to regular screenings, and he received a combination of targeted radiation therapy and hormone therapy. These treatments were more refined and effective, with fewer side effects. My father responded well to the treatment and has been in remission for several years.

As for me, Rosenthal Arnold, my family's history has made me acutely aware of the importance of early detection and proactive health management. I regularly undergo screenings and maintain a healthy lifestyle to mitigate my risk. Advances in medical research and treatment options give me hope that, if I were to face a similar diagnosis, my outcome would be far more positive than that of my grandfather.

Our family's experience with prostate cancer underscores the critical importance of early detection, advancements in medical research, and the evolution of treatment options. It is a journey marked by pain and loss, but also by hope and resilience as we continue to navigate the legacy of prostate cancer within our family.

Dr. Ben and I continued writing about prostate cancer, and our fourth book became more focused on cancer overall. Titled "The Complete Guide to Surviving Prostate Cancer: A Journey of Hope and Healing," the book offers increasingly positive news, especially in the chapters on advanced and metastatic prostate cancer. From my dad's and my own experiences, we've learned the importance of early diagnosis and treatment. Our hope is that prostate cancer will become a minor issue, caught early, treated effectively, and then life goes on as normal.

Within these pages lies not just our narrative, but a lifeline—a guide illuminating the path for those navigating the treacherous waters of prostate cancer. Let our journey be your beacon, guiding you through the darkest nights to the dawn of healing and renewal.

Join us, as we embark on a journey of resilience, healing, and above all, hope. This is not just a book—it is a testament to the indomitable spirit of the human heart.

CHAPTER 1: Understanding the Prostate: A Crash Course in Male Anatomy

<u>CHAPTER OUTLINE:</u>

Understanding the Prostate: A Crash Course in Male Anatomy

- Location of the Prostate
- Anatomy of the Male Genital Organ
- Prostate Gland Connection with other Genital Organs such as:
    - Seminal Vesicle
    - Testes
    - Urethra
- Anatomy of the Prostate Gland

☐ The Role and Function of the Prostate

LOCATION OF THE PROSTATE

The prostate gland, often referred to simply as the prostate, is a crucial component of the male reproductive system. Situated just below the bladder and in front of the rectum, it is roughly the size of a walnut and surrounds the urethra, the tube responsible for carrying urine and semen out of the body. Despite its small size, the prostate plays a vital role in both urinary and sexual function.

Anatomy of the Male Genitalia:

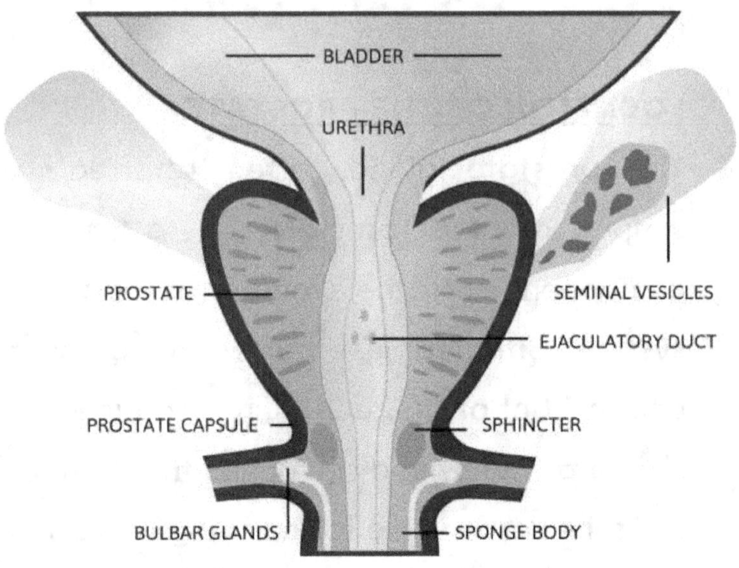

ANATOMY OF THE MALE GENITAL ORGAN

To fully comprehend the significance of the prostate, it's essential to first understand the anatomy of the male genitalia. At the base of the penis lies the root of the penis, which extends internally to form the penile shaft. Encased within the penile shaft are three cylindrical structures known as the corpora cavernosa and the corpus spongiosum. These tissues are responsible for the erectile function of the penis, allowing it to become erect during sexual arousal.

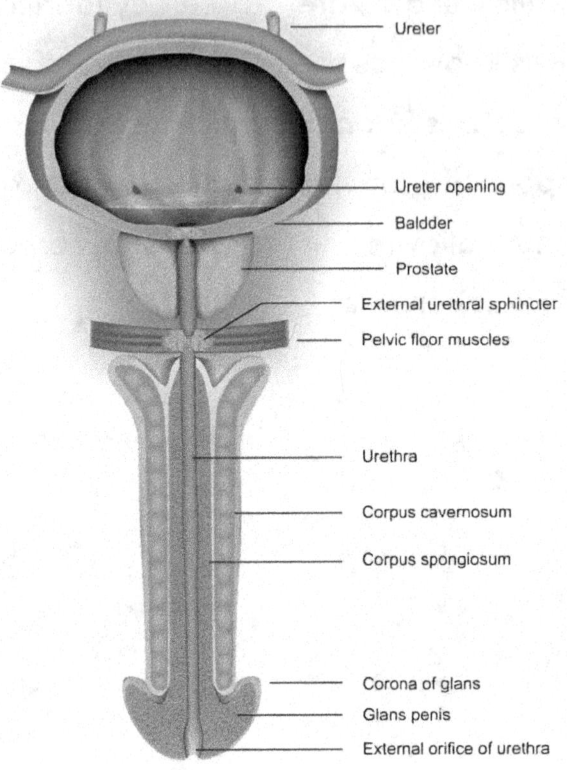

Connection with Other Genital Organs:

The prostate gland is intricately connected to several other organs within the male genitalia, forming a complex network that facilitates reproductive function.

1. Seminal Vesicles: Positioned above the prostate gland, the seminal vesicles are responsible for producing the majority of the fluid that makes up semen. During ejaculation, seminal fluid from the seminal vesicles combines with sperm from the testes and prostatic fluid from the prostate gland to form semen.

2. Testes: The primary male reproductive organs, the testes are responsible for producing sperm and testosterone, the male sex hormone. Sperm produced in the testes travel through the epididymis and vas deferens before reaching the seminal vesicles and prostate gland for ejaculation.

3. Urethra: The urethra serves as a conduit for both urine and semen, allowing for the passage of fluids out of the body. It runs through the center of the prostate gland

and is surrounded by prostatic tissue, which can become enlarged due to conditions such as BPH or prostate cancer, leading to urinary symptoms.

Male Reproductive System

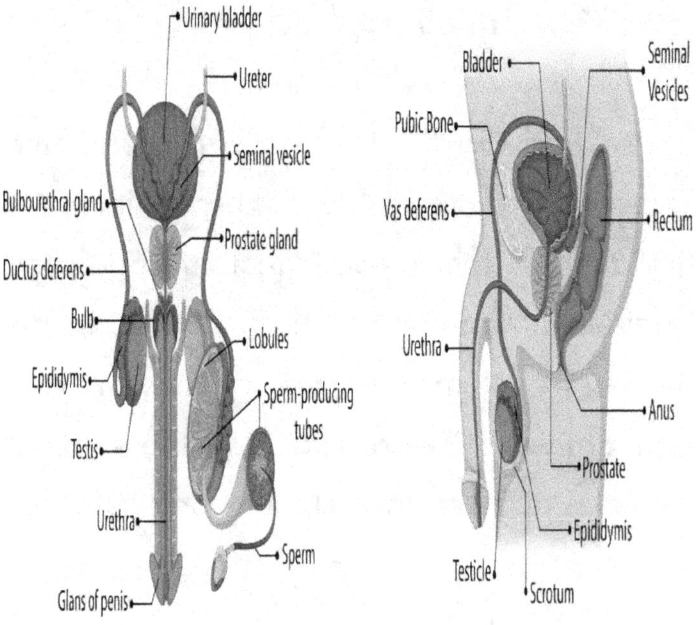

1. Prostate Gland: The walnut-shaped gland located beneath the bladder and surrounding the urethra.

2. Urethra: The tube that carries urine from the bladder and semen from the reproductive organs out of the body.

3. Bladder: The organ that stores urine before it is excreted.

4. Seminal Vesicles: Glands located behind the bladder that produce additional seminal fluid to mix with sperm.

5. Vas Deferens: Tubes that transport sperm from the testes to the seminal vesicles during ejaculation.

6. Testicles: Male reproductive organs responsible for producing sperm and testosterone.

7. Rectum: The final section of the large intestine, located behind the prostate gland.

8. Penis: Male external organ involved in sexual intercourse and urination.

ANATOMY OF THE PROSTATE GLAND:

The prostate gland is often likened to the size and shape of a walnut, although its dimensions may vary slightly among individuals. It consists of several distinct regions, each serving a specific function in the reproductive process.

1. Peripheral Zone: The largest portion of the prostate gland, comprising approximately 70-80% of its volume, is known as the peripheral zone. This region is located at the back of the gland and is the most common site for prostate cancer to develop.

2. Central Zone: Situated at the base of the prostate gland, the central zone surrounds the ejaculatory ducts, through which semen travels from the seminal vesicles to the urethra. Despite its smaller size compared to the peripheral zone, the central zone plays a crucial role in seminal fluid production.

3. Transition Zone: The transition zone lies adjacent to the urethra and accounts for approximately 5-10% of the prostate gland's volume. It is primarily responsible for the growth of the prostate gland during puberty and can be a site of benign prostatic hyperplasia (BPH) in older men, leading to urinary symptoms such as hesitancy and urgency.

4. Anterior Fibromuscular Stroma: Surrounding the transition zone and peripheral zone is the anterior fibromuscular stroma, a dense layer of connective tissue and smooth muscle fibers. This structural framework provides support to the prostate gland and helps maintain its integrity.

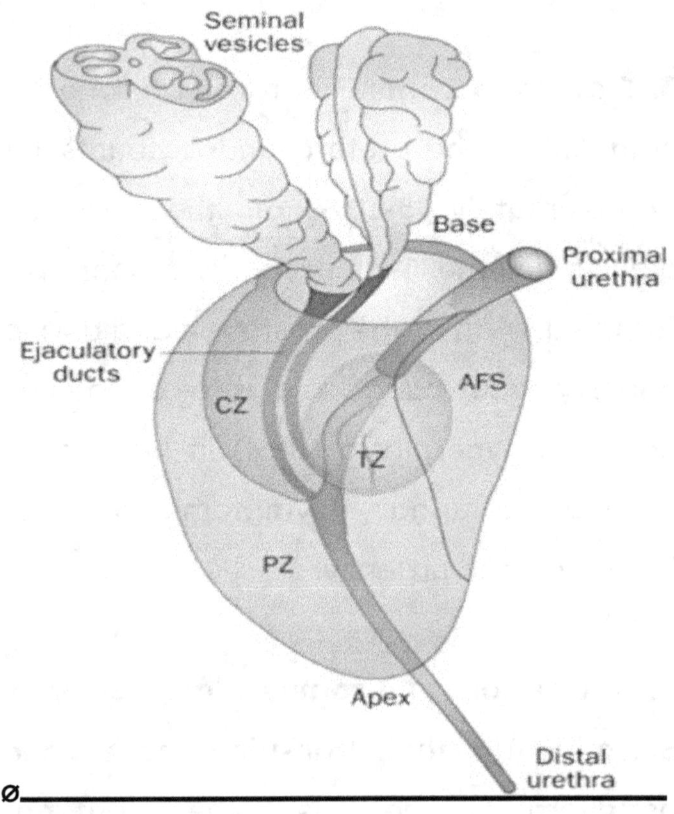

Anterior Fibromuscular Zone (AFZ):

Peripheral Zone: (PZ)

Central Zone (CZ):

Transition Zone (TZ):

THE ROLE OF THE PROSTATE:

The prostate gland is nestled between the bladder and the rectum, with its base resting against the bladder neck and its apex extending towards the urogenital diaphragm. Its strategic location enables the prostate to perform several crucial functions:

Function of the Prostate:

The primary function of the prostate gland is to produce seminal fluid, a milky substance that nourishes and transports sperm during ejaculation. This fluid, comprising enzymes, proteins, and other substances, provides the optimal environment for sperm survival and motility.

1. Production of Prostatic Fluid: The prostate gland secretes a milky fluid rich in enzymes, proteins, and minerals, which constitutes a significant portion of seminal fluid. This prostatic fluid serves as a nutrient source for sperm, enhances their motility, and helps neutralize the acidity of the vaginal environment, thus promoting sperm survival and fertility.

2. Contribution to Ejaculation: During sexual arousal, the prostate contracts rhythmically, releasing its prostatic fluid into the urethra. This mixture of prostatic fluid, sperm from the testes, and secretions from the seminal vesicles forms semen, which is expelled from the body during ejaculation.

3. Regulation of Urinary Function: The prostate gland surrounds the urethra, acting as a muscular sphincter to control the flow of urine. It contracts during ejaculation to prevent urine from mixing with semen and relaxes during urination to allow the passage of urine through the urethra.

In summary, the prostate gland is a multifaceted organ integral to male reproductive and urinary health. Its anatomical location and physiological functions underscore its importance in both sexual function and overall well-being. Understanding the role of the prostate lays the foundation for comprehending the complexities of prostate cancer and the implications of its diagnosis and treatment

CHAPTER 2: Unveiling the Causes of Prostate Cancer and Strategies for Prevention

CHAPTER OUTLINE

UNVEILING THE CAUSES OF PROSTATE CANCER

1) Age: Aging promotes prostate cancer through:
   - Accumulation of genetic mutations,
   - Hormonal changes at old age
   - Inflammation and Oxidative Stress due to aging
   - Telomere Shortening and cellular senescene as a result of aging

- Epigenetic Alterations occur at old age
- Alter immune function: at old age, immunity is weaken

2) Family History: Members of the same family has tendency to have prostate cancer in common due to:

- Genetic Predisposition
- Shared Environmental Exposures
- Hormonal Influence
- Shared Screening Practices
- Epigenetic Modifications
- Gene-Environment interactions

3) Race and Ethnicity: Comparison in Prostate Cancer incidence rates among races :

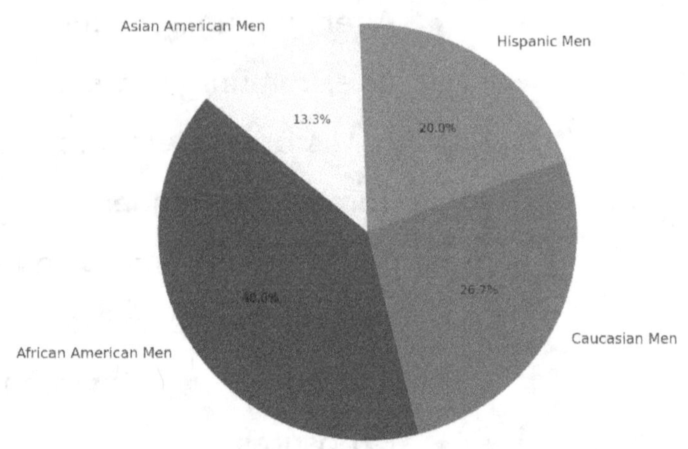

Here is the pie chart showing the relative incidence rates of prostate cancer among different racial groups, with the specified colors:

- African American Men: Blue➡️ 40%

- Caucasian Men: Green➡️ 26.7%

- Hispanic Men: Red➡️ 20.0%

-Asian American Men:Yellow.➡☐ 13.3%

mechanisms behind these disparities involves:

☐ Genetics Variations

☐ Biological Factors

☐ Environmental Exposures

☐ Socio-Economic Factors

☐ Healthcare Disparities

4. Genetics

- Inherited Genetic Mutations such as BRCA1 and BRCA2 genes
- Family History : Genetic make up of members of the same family consist of Prostate Cancer as one of the traits and characteristics that runs in the family.

- Polygenic Risk Scores: the total number of genetic variants that an individual has to assess their heritable risk of developing a particular disease

- Tumor Suppressor Genes and Oncogenes: Mutations or deletions in Tumor Suppressor Genes such as PTEN and TP53 can disrupt their function, allowing uncontrolled cell proliferation and tumor formation.

- Androgen Receptor Signalling: Genetic variations in Androgen Receptor gene can promote initiation and progression of prostate cancer

5. Lifestyle factors: Several lifestyle habit promote prostate cancer development and

progression. This habit or lifestyle factors are:

- Diet: Excessive intake of saturated fats
- Obesity
- Sedentary lifestyle or inadequate physical activity
- Alcohol consumption
- Smoking
- Exposure to harmful chemicals

PREVENTIVE STRATEGIES FOR PROSTATE CANCER

- ☐ Avoid Exposure to Harmful Chemicals
- ☐ Adopting a healthy lifestyle:
  - Healthy Diet
  - Regular Exercise
  - Maintain a Healthy Weight
  - Limit Alcohol Consumption

- Regular Screening:

UNVEILING THE CAUSES OF PROSTATE CANCER

Prostate cancer is one of the most prevalent forms of cancer among men worldwide, with millions of new cases diagnosed each year. While the exact cause of prostate cancer remains unknown, researchers have identified several risk factors and potential contributors to its development. In this chapter, we will explore the multifaceted nature of prostate cancer etiology and delve into strategies for prevention and risk reduction.

Understanding Risk Factors:

1. Age:

Age is the single most significant risk factor for prostate cancer, with the disease predominantly affecting men over the age of 50. As men grow older, the risk of developing prostate cancer increases exponentially, making regular screening and early detection crucial for older individuals.

Bio-mechanism

Age is one of the most significant risk factors for prostate cancer, with the majority of cases occurring in men over the age of 65. Understanding the mechanisms by which age contributes to the development of prostate cancer involves examining various biological and environmental factors that change with age.

A) Accumulation of Genetic Mutations:

As men age, their cells undergo cumulative genetic alterations due to factors such as DNA replication errors, exposure to environmental carcinogens, and impaired DNA repair mechanisms. These genetic mutations can accumulate over time, leading to the development of prostate cancer. Mutations in genes involved in cell growth regulation, such as tumor suppressor genes and oncogenes, can disrupt normal cellular processes and promote the uncontrolled growth of prostate cells.

B). Hormonal Changes:

Aging is associated with alterations in hormone levels, including changes in testosterone and other androgens, which play a critical role in prostate cancer development and progression. While prostate cancer is typically androgen-dependent in its early stages, aging is associated with an increase in the prevalence of castration-resistant prostate cancer (CRPC), which may be driven by alterations in androgen receptor signaling pathways and the emergence of androgen-independent tumor clones.

C. Inflammation and Oxidative Stress:

Aging is characterized by chronic inflammation and increased oxidative stress, which can contribute to DNA damage, cellular dysfunction, and inflammation-mediated carcinogenesis. In the prostate gland, chronic inflammation, often associated with conditions such as prostatitis or benign prostatic hyperplasia (BPH), can create a pro-carcinogenic microenvironment conducive to the development and progression of prostate cancer.

D) Telomere Shortening and Cellular Senescence:

Telomeres, protective caps at the ends of chromosomes, undergo shortening with each cell division, eventually reaching a critical length that triggers cellular senescence or apoptosis (programmed cell death). Aging is associated with telomere attrition and the accumulation of senescent cells, which can promote inflammation, tissue remodeling, and tumor progression in the prostate gland.

E) Epigenetic Alterations:

Epigenetic modifications, including DNA methylation, histone modifications, and non-coding RNA regulation, play a crucial role in gene expression regulation and chromatin remodeling. Age-related changes in epigenetic patterns can influence the expression of genes involved in prostate cancer development and progression, potentially contributing to the age-associated increase in prostate cancer risk.

UNVEILING THE CAUSES OF PROSTATE CANCER

F) Altered Immune Function:
Aging is associated with immune system dysregulation, including immunosenescence (age-related decline in immune function) and chronic low-grade inflammation (inflammaging). These changes can impair immune surveillance and tumor immune responses, allowing for

the escape and proliferation of malignant cells in the prostate gland.

☐ Agee-related changes in genetic, hormonal, inflammatory, oxidative, and epigenetic processes contribute to the increased risk of prostate cancer in older men. Understanding these mechanisms can inform strategies for early detection, prevention, and treatment of prostate cancer in aging populations. Regular screening, lifestyle modifications, and targeted therapies tailored to the aging prostate microenvironment may help mitigate the impact of age as a risk factor for prostate cancer.

2. Family History:

A family history of prostate cancer significantly elevates an individual's risk of developing the disease. Men with a first-degree relative (father, brother) who has been diagnosed with prostate cancer are at higher risk, particularly if the relative was diagnosed at a young age or had an aggressive form of the disease.

Bio-mechanism

A. Genetic Predisposition:

Sometimes, certain genes that we inherit from our family members can make us more likely to get prostate cancer. So, if someone in your family has had prostate cancer, you might have inherited these genes, which could increase your risk of getting the disease too.

B. Shared Environmental Exposures:

We often live in similar environments and have similar habits to our family members. If we're exposed to things that can cause cancer, like certain chemicals or unhealthy habits, our family members might also be exposed to them, which can raise the risk for everyone in the family.

C. Hormonal Influence:

Hormones, which are natural chemicals in our bodies, can affect prostate cancer risk. If other family members have had cancers that are affected by hormones, like breast cancer in women, it might suggest that hormonal factors could also affect prostate cancer risk in men in the family.

D. Shared Screening Practices:

Families often have similar habits when it comes to going to the doctor for check-ups. If one family member gets screened for prostate cancer regularly and finds it early, others in the family might also do the same, which could lead to more cases being found within the family.

E. Epigenetic Modifications:

Sometimes, our genes can be affected by things in our environment, like what we eat or where we live. These changes, called epigenetic changes, can affect how our genes work and might increase the risk of prostate cancer, especially if they run in the family.

UNVEILING THE CAUSES OF PROSTATE CANCER

F. Gene-Environment Interactions:

Our genes can interact with things in our environment, like what we're exposed to or how we live. This interaction between our genes and our environment can affect our risk of getting prostate cancer, and if it runs in the family, it's important to consider both genetic and environmental factors when thinking about the risk.

3. Race and Ethnicity:

Prostate cancer exhibits significant racial and ethnic disparities, with African American men facing the highest incidence rates and mortality rates globally. Asian American and Hispanic men have lower rates of prostate cancer compared to Caucasians but may still be at risk, particularly if they have other predisposing factors. Prostate cancer affects different racial and ethnic groups in different ways. Let's break it down:

African American Men: African American men have the highest rates of prostate cancer in the world. Not only are they more likely to get prostate cancer, but they also tend to have more aggressive forms of the disease. This means it can be harder to treat, leading to higher mortality rates.

Caucasian Men: Caucasian men have a higher risk of prostate cancer compared to some other groups, but it's not as high as African American men. However, it's still important for Caucasian men to be aware of the risk and get regular screenings, especially as they get older.

Asian American Men: Asian American men generally have lower rates of prostate cancer compared to African American and Caucasian men. However, this doesn't mean they're completely safe. They should still be aware of the risk and talk to their doctor about screening, especially if they have other risk factors.

Hispanic Men: Hispanic men also have lower rates of prostate cancer compared to African American and Caucasian men. However, like Asian American men, they should still pay attention to their risk and talk to their doctor about screening if they have other risk factors.

Overall, it's important for all men, regardless of their race or ethnicity, to be aware of the risk of prostate cancer and to talk to their doctor about screening options. Early detection can save lives, so don't hesitate to ask your doctor about prostate cancer screening, especially as you get older.

Race and ethnicity are significant risk factors for prostate cancer, with notable differences in incidence and mortality rates among different racial and ethnic groups. Understanding the mechanisms behind these disparities involves exploring a combination of genetic, biological, environmental, and socio-economic factors.

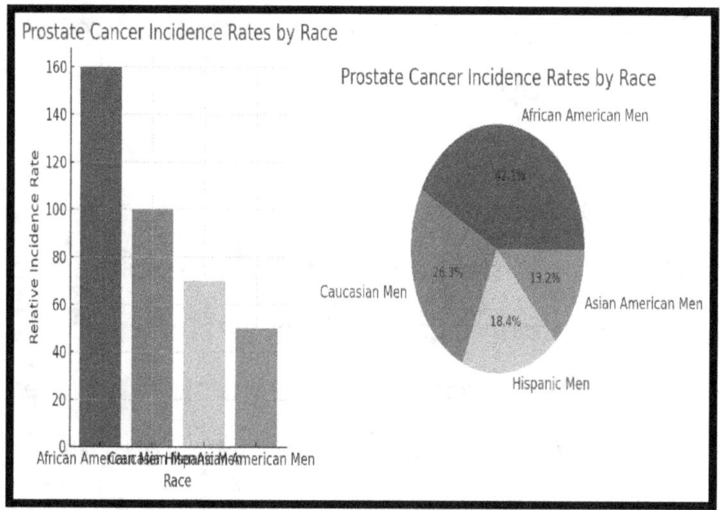

Here are the bar chart and pie chart comparing the incidence rates of prostate cancer among different racial groups:

-Bar Chart: This shows the relative incidence rates with African American men having the highest rate, followed by

Caucasian men, Hispanic men, and Asian American men.

- Pie Chart: This visualizes the proportion of prostate cancer incidence rates among the races, highlighting the higher incidence in African American men compared to the other groups.

A. Genetic Variations:

Genetic differences among racial and ethnic groups can influence susceptibility to prostate cancer. For example, studies have identified certain genetic mutations, such as variations in the BRCA1 and BRCA2 genes, that are more prevalent in certain populations and are associated with an increased risk of prostate cancer. African-American men, in particular, have been found to have a higher prevalence of these genetic mutations compared to men of other racial and ethnic backgrounds.

B. Biological Factors:

Biological differences in the prostate gland and hormonal profiles may contribute to racial disparities in prostate cancer risk. For instance, African-American men tend to have larger prostate glands and higher levels of certain hormones, such as testosterone, which have been associated with an increased risk of prostate cancer. Additionally, differences in tumor biology and aggressiveness may play a role in the observed disparities, with some studies suggesting that prostate cancers in African-American men are more likely to be diagnosed at later stages and to be more aggressive compared to those in other racial and ethnic groups.

C. Environmental Exposures:

Environmental factors, including exposure to carcinogens and pollutants, may contribute to racial disparities in prostate cancer risk. For example, studies have shown that African-American men are more likely to be exposed to certain environmental toxins, such as cadmium and polycyclic aromatic hydrocarbons (PAHs), which have been linked to an increased risk of prostate cancer. Occupational exposures, dietary habits, and lifestyle factors may also vary among racial and ethnic groups and contribute to differences in prostate cancer risk.

D. Socio-Economic Factors:

Socio-economic factors, including access to healthcare, socioeconomic status, and health behaviors, can impact prostate cancer risk and outcomes. African-American men, as well as men from other minority racial and ethnic groups, are more likely to experience disparities in access to healthcare, leading to delays in diagnosis, suboptimal treatment, and poorer outcomes. Additionally, socio-economic factors such as poverty, limited education, and lack of health insurance may contribute to disparities in prostate cancer risk factors such as obesity, smoking, and dietary habits.

E. Healthcare Disparities:

Disparities in healthcare access, utilization, and quality of care contribute significantly to the observed differences in prostate cancer outcomes among racial and ethnic groups. African-American men are less likely to undergo routine screening for prostate cancer and are more likely to be diagnosed with advanced-stage disease, leading to higher mortality rates compared to men of other racial and ethnic backgrounds. Additionally, disparities in treatment options, adherence to treatment guidelines, and access to clinical trials may further exacerbate the disparities in prostate cancer outcomes.

□□ The mechanisms underlying the association between race and ethnicity and prostate cancer risk are complex and multifactorial, involving a combination of genetic, biological, environmental, socio-economic, and healthcare-related factors. Addressing these disparities requires a comprehensive approach that includes efforts to improve access to healthcare, promote early detection and screening, reduce exposure to environmental carcinogens, and address social determinants of health.

4. Genetics:

Genetics play a big role in prostate cancer. Think of genes as instructions that tell our bodies how to work. Sometimes, these instructions can have mistakes, called mutations. Certain genes, like BRCA1 and BRCA2, are famous for their role in breast and ovarian cancer, but they can also affect prostate cancer risk. Imagine these genes as guardians protecting our cells. When they work properly, they repair any damage and keep cells from growing out of control. But if they have mutations, they might not do their job well, making it easier for cancer to develop. It's not just BRCA genes; there are other genes too, all doing similar jobs. They help with repairing DNA and keeping cell growth in check. When these genes have variations or mutations, they can increase the chances of getting prostate cancer.

So, in simple terms, genetics can affect prostate cancer risk by causing mutations in specific genes that normally keep our cells healthy and prevent them from turning into cancer. Genetics plays a significant role in prostate cancer risk, with numerous studies highlighting the strong influence of inherited genetic factors on the development of the disease.

Bio-mechanism

Understanding the mechanisms through which genetics contribute to prostate cancer risk is essential for identifying individuals at higher risk and developing targeted prevention and treatment strategies. These mechanisms are;

A. Inherited Genetic Mutations: One of the most direct mechanisms linking genetics to prostate cancer risk is the inheritance of specific genetic mutations.

Mutations in certain genes, such as BRCA1 and BRCA2, have been associated with an increased risk of prostate cancer. These genes are involved in repairing damaged DNA and maintaining genomic stability. When mutations occur in these genes, DNA repair mechanisms may be compromised, leading to an accumulation of genetic alterations and an increased risk of cancer development.

B. Family History:

Family history is a well-established risk factor for prostate cancer, with individuals who have a first-degree relative (such as a father or brother) diagnosed with the disease at higher risk. While part of this increased risk may be due to shared environmental factors, such as lifestyle and dietary habits, genetic factors also play a significant role. Familial clustering of prostate cancer suggests the presence of shared genetic susceptibility factors within families, further supporting the genetic basis of the disease.

C.. Polygenic Risk Scores: Prostate cancer is a complex disease influenced by multiple genetic variants across the genome. Recent advances in genomic research have led to the development of polygenic risk scores (PRS), which combine information from numerous genetic variants to estimate an individual's genetic predisposition to prostate cancer. Genome-wide association studies (GWAS) have identified hundreds of common genetic variants associated with prostate cancer risk. These variants may individually confer only a modest increase in risk, but their cumulative effects can substantially elevate the overall risk of developing the disease.

D. Tumor Suppressor Genes and Oncogenes: Genetic alterations affecting tumor suppressor genes and oncogenes can contribute to prostate cancer initiation and progression. Tumor suppressor genes, such as PTEN and TP53, normally regulate cell growth and prevent the development of cancer by repairing damaged DNA or inducing cell death (apoptosis) in abnormal cells. Mutations or deletions in these genes can disrupt their function, allowing uncontrolled cell proliferation and tumor formation. Similarly, oncogenes, such as MYC and ERG, promote cell growth and division when activated by genetic alterations like amplifications or translocations. Dysregulation of these genes can drive prostate cancer development by enhancing cell proliferation and survival.

E. Androgen Receptor Signaling: Androgen receptor (AR) signaling plays a crucial role in prostate cancer development and progression. Genetic variations in genes involved in the androgen signaling pathway, including the AR gene itself, can influence individual susceptibility to prostate cancer. Polymorphisms in the AR gene may affect androgen receptor function, altering the responsiveness of prostate cells to androgen stimulation and promoting tumor growth. Additionally, somatic mutations in the AR gene can confer resistance to androgen deprivation therapy, a common treatment for advanced prostate cancer, leading to treatment failure and disease progression.

☐ Overall, genetics contribute significantly to prostate cancer risk through various mechanisms, including inherited genetic mutations, family history, polygenic inheritance, alterations in tumor suppressor genes and oncogenes, and dysregulation of androgen receptor signaling. Understanding these genetic factors can inform risk assessment, screening strategies, and personalized treatment approaches for individuals at increased risk of prostate cancer.

UNVEILING THE CAUSES OF PROSTATE CANCER

5. Lifestyle Factors:

Several lifestyle factors have been linked to prostate cancer risk, including diet, obesity, and physical activity. A diet high in saturated fats and red meat and low in fruits, vegetables, and fiber may increase the risk of prostate cancer, while regular exercise and weight management can help reduce risk. Lifestyle choices can greatly affect your risk of prostate cancer. Here's a breakdown of how certain habits can impact your chances of developing this disease:

1. Diet: What you eat plays a big role. Foods high in saturated fats, like fatty meats and dairy products, as well as red meat, have been linked to a higher risk of prostate cancer. On the other hand, a diet rich in fruits, vegetables, and fiber can help lower your risk. Try to include more plant-based foods in your meals and limit your intake of fatty and processed foods.

<u>High consumption of red and processed meats</u>: Red and processed meats contain carcinogens, such as heterocyclic amines (HCAs) and polycyclic aromatic hydrocarbons (PAHs), formed during cooking at high temperatures. These compounds may promote the development of prostate cancer by causing DNA damage and increasing inflammation.

<u>Low intake of fruits and vegetables:</u> Fruits and vegetables are rich in antioxidants, vitamins, and minerals that help protect against cancer by neutralizing free radicals and reducing inflammation. A diet lacking in these protective nutrients may increase the risk of prostate cancer.

2. Obesity: Being overweight or obese can increase your risk of prostate cancer. Extra body fat, especially around your waistline, can lead to inflammation and hormonal changes that may promote the growth of cancer cells. Maintaining a healthy weight through proper diet and regular exercise is important for reducing your risk.

Break it down!

- ☐ Obesity is associated with chronic inflammation and altered levels of hormones such as insulin and insulin-like growth factor 1 (IGF-1), which can promote the growth and progression of prostate cancer cells.

- ☐ Adipose tissue (fat cells) can produce hormones and cytokines that stimulate cell growth and angiogenesis (formation of new blood vessels), creating an environment conducive to tumor growth.

- Obesity is also linked to insulin resistance and elevated levels of insulin and insulin-like growth factor 1 (IGF-1), which may promote the growth and proliferation of prostate cancer cells.

3. Physical Activity: Regular exercise is not only good for your overall health but can also lower your risk of prostate cancer. Aim for at least 30 minutes of moderate to vigorous exercise most days of the week. Activities like brisk walking, cycling, swimming, or jogging can help keep your weight in check and reduce inflammation in your body, lowering your risk of cancer.

- Regular physical activity helps maintain a healthy weight and reduces inflammation, insulin resistance, and levels of circulating hormones such as insulin and IGF-1, which may inhibit the development and progression of prostate cancer.

☐ Exercise may also have direct anti-cancer effects by enhancing immune function, promoting DNA repair, and reducing oxidative stress and inflammation.

4. Alcohol Consumption:

- Heavy alcohol consumption can increase the risk of prostate cancer through various mechanisms, including the metabolism of ethanol into acetaldehyde, a known carcinogen.

- Alcohol may also interfere with the body's ability to absorb and utilize essential nutrients, such as folate and vitamin D, which play important roles in cancer prevention.

Chronic alcohol consumption is known to cause inflammation, which is a recognized factor in cancer development. Inflammation can promote genetic mutations and alterations in the prostate, fostering an environment conducive to cancer growth.

5. Smoking:

Smoking is not only a risk factor for lung cancer but may also increase the risk of developing aggressive prostate cancer. Tobacco smoke contains numerous carcinogens that can damage DNA and promote tumor growth. Smoking is also associated with inflammation and oxidative stress, which can contribute to cancer development.

Smoking and Prostate Cancer: Understanding the Risks

While smoking is most commonly associated with lung cancer, it is also a significant risk factor for various other cancers, including aggressive forms of prostate cancer. The harmful effects of tobacco smoke extend beyond the respiratory system, influencing cellular processes and contributing to carcinogenesis in multiple organs. This detailed examination explores how smoking increases the risk of aggressive prostate cancer, focusing on the carcinogenic compounds in tobacco smoke, the biological mechanisms involved, and the broader implications for men's health.

Carcinogens in Tobacco Smoke

Tobacco smoke contains over 7,000 chemicals, with at least 70 known carcinogens. These harmful substances include:

1. Polycyclic Aromatic Hydrocarbons (PAHs)

- **Mechanism**: PAHs can form DNA adducts, which are complexes that directly attach to DNA, causing mutations. These mutations can disrupt normal cell function and promote the development of cancer.

2. Nitrosamines:

- Mechanism: Nitrosamines, particularly N-nitrosonornicotine (NNN) and 4-(methylnitrosamino)-1-(3-pyridyl)-1-butanone (NNK), are potent carcinogens. They induce genetic mutations by forming adducts with DNA bases, leading to miscoding during DNA replication.

3. Formaldehyde:

-Formaldehyde can cause DNA-protein cross-links and chromosomal aberrations, interfering with DNA repair mechanisms and promoting carcinogenesis.

4. Cadmium:

- Mechanism: This heavy metal is a known carcinogen that can induce oxidative stress and disrupt DNA repair processes, increasing the risk of mutations.

UNVEILING THE CAUSES OF PROSTATE CANCER

Biological Mechanisms Linking Smoking to Prostate Cancer

The carcinogens in tobacco smoke initiate and promote cancer development through several interconnected biological mechanisms:

1. DNA Damage and Mutations:

- Carcinogens in tobacco smoke can directly damage DNA, leading to mutations that disrupt normal cellular function. These mutations can activate oncogenes (genes that promote cell proliferation) or inactivate tumor suppressor genes (genes that prevent uncontrolled cell growth), facilitating cancer development.

2. Oxidative Stress

- Smoking generates high levels of reactive oxygen species (ROS), which cause oxidative stress. ROS can damage cellular components, including lipids, proteins, and DNA, leading to mutations and promoting tumorigenesis. Chronic oxidative stress also contributes to an inflammatory environment, further enhancing cancer risk.

3. Inflammation

- Tobacco smoke induces a chronic inflammatory response, characterized by the release of cytokines and other inflammatory mediators. Chronic inflammation can promote a microenvironment conducive to cancer development by enhancing cell proliferation, inhibiting apoptosis (programmed cell death), and increasing angiogenesis (formation of new blood vessels that supply tumors).

4. Immune Suppression:

- Smoking can impair the immune system's ability to detect and eliminate cancerous cells. By weakening immune surveillance, smoking allows abnormal cells to evade immune detection and grow uncontrollably.

Evidence Linking Smoking to Aggressive Prostate Cancer

Several epidemiological studies and meta-analyses have demonstrated a link between smoking and an increased risk of aggressive prostate cancer:

1. Increased Risk of High-Grade Prostate Cancer

- Studies have found that smokers are more likely to develop high-grade prostate cancer, which is more aggressive and has a poorer prognosis compared to low-grade forms. High-grade prostate cancers are characterized by higher Gleason scores, indicating more abnormal and rapidly proliferating cells.

2. Higher Mortality Rates:

- Smokers diagnosed with prostate cancer have higher mortality rates compared to non-smokers. This is partly due to the increased likelihood of developing aggressive tumors and partly due to the overall detrimental effects of smoking on health, which can complicate cancer treatment and recovery.

UNVEILING THE CAUSES OF PROSTATE CANCER

3. Recurrence and Progression:

- Smoking is associated with a higher risk of cancer recurrence and progression after treatment. Smokers who undergo prostate cancer treatment, such as surgery or radiation therapy, are more likely to experience a return of the disease compared to non-smokers.

Broader Implications for Men's Health

The impact of smoking on prostate cancer risk highlights the broader health implications of tobacco use:

1. Comorbid Conditions:

- Smokers are at increased risk for various comorbid conditions, including cardiovascular disease, respiratory illnesses, and other cancers. These conditions can complicate the management and treatment of prostate cancer, leading to worse outcomes.

2. Impact on Treatment Efficacy:

- Smoking can affect the efficacy of prostate cancer treatments. For example, it can impair wound healing after surgery and reduce the effectiveness of radiation therapy by promoting hypoxia (low oxygen levels) in tissues, which makes cancer cells more resistant to radiation.

3. Quality of Life

- The cumulative health effects of smoking can significantly diminish quality of life. Chronic diseases, reduced physical fitness, and complications from cancer treatment can all contribute to a lower quality of life for smokers.

Smoking is a well-established risk factor for numerous cancers, including aggressive prostate cancer. The carcinogenic compounds in tobacco smoke damage DNA, induce oxidative stress, promote inflammation, and impair immune function, all of which contribute to cancer development and progression. Given the significant health risks, smoking cessation is a critical step for reducing the risk of prostate cancer and improving overall health. Public health initiatives and personal efforts to quit smoking can profoundly impact individual and community health outcomes, underscoring the importance of addressing tobacco use in cancer prevention strategies.

6. Exposure to Harmful Chemicals:

- Occupational exposure to certain chemicals, such as cadmium, pesticides, herbicides, and industrial pollutants, may increase the risk of prostate cancer.

- These chemicals can disrupt hormone balance, damage DNA, and promote inflammation and oxidative stress, all of which can contribute to prostate cancer development.

Exposure to Harmful Chemicals and Prostate Cancer Risk

Occupational and environmental exposure to harmful chemicals is important but often under-appreciated risk factor for various cancers, including prostate cancer. Certain chemicals, such as cadmium, pesticides, herbicides, industrial pollutants, and Agent Orange, have been linked to an increased risk of prostate cancer. Understanding the mechanisms by which these chemicals affect the body and contribute to carcinogenesis is crucial for prevention and risk mitigation.

Key Harmful Chemicals Linked to Prostate Cancer:

1. Cadmium:

Cadmium is a heavy metal found in industrial workplaces, such as battery manufacturing, metal smelting, and plastics production. It can also be present in cigarette smoke.

- **Mechanism of Action:** Cadmium is known to disrupt hormone balance by mimicking estrogen, leading to hormonal dysregulation. It can also cause direct DNA damage and interfere with DNA repair mechanisms. Additionally, cadmium induces oxidative stress and chronic inflammation, creating an environment conducive to cancer development.

UNVEILING THE CAUSES OF PROSTATE CANCER

2. Pesticides:

Pesticides are chemicals used in agriculture to protect crops from pests and diseases. Farmers, agricultural workers, and individuals living near agricultural areas are at higher risk of exposure.

- **Mechanism of Action:** Many pesticides are endocrine disruptors, meaning they can interfere with hormone function. They can alter the levels and activity of hormones like androgens and estrogens, which are critical in prostate cancer development. Pesticides also induce oxidative stress and inflammation, which can lead to DNA damage and increased cancer risk.

3. Herbicides:

Herbicides are chemicals used to control unwanted plants (weeds). Similar to pesticides, they are commonly used in agriculture and landscaping.

- **Mechanism of Action::** Some herbicides act as endocrine disruptors, interfering with normal hormonal signaling. They can also generate reactive oxygen species (ROS), leading to oxidative stress and DNA damage. Chronic exposure can result in persistent inflammation and cellular changes that promote cancer.

4. Industrial Pollutants:

Industrial pollutants include a wide range of chemicals released from manufacturing processes, such as polychlorinated biphenyls (PCBs), dioxins, and solvents.

- **Mechanism of Action:** These pollutants can disrupt endocrine function, generate oxidative stress, and cause inflammation. Many industrial chemicals are also genotoxic, meaning they directly damage DNA and interfere with cellular repair processes, increasing the risk of cancer development.

5. Agent Orange:

Agent Orange is a herbicide and defoliant chemical used extensively during the Vietnam War. It contains dioxin, a highly toxic compound.

- **Mechanism of Action**: Agent Orange, particularly its dioxin component, is a potent endocrine disruptor and carcinogen. Dioxin can interfere with hormone signaling, induce oxidative stress, and cause chronic inflammation. It can also directly damage DNA and impair the body's ability to repair genetic material, significantly increasing the risk of developing aggressive prostate cancer.

Mechanisms Linking Harmful Chemicals to Prostate Cancer

1. Hormonal Disruption:

- **Endocrine Disruptors:** Chemicals like cadmium, certain pesticides, herbicides, and dioxins in Agent Orange can mimic or block natural hormones, disrupting the endocrine system. This disruption can alter the levels of hormones such as testosterone and estrogen, which play critical roles in the growth and function of prostate cells. Hormonal imbalances can stimulate the proliferation of prostate cells and increase the likelihood of malignant transformation.

UNVEILING THE CAUSES OF PROSTATE CANCER

2. DNA Damage:

- **Genotoxicity**: Many harmful chemicals are genotoxic, meaning they can cause direct damage to DNA. This damage can result in mutations, deletions, and chromosomal abnormalities. When the DNA repair mechanisms are overwhelmed or impaired, these genetic alterations can accumulate, leading to cancer development.

3. Oxidative Stress:

- **Reactive Oxygen Species (ROS):** Chemicals like cadmium, industrial pollutants, and components of Agent Orange can generate ROS, which cause oxidative stress. ROS are highly reactive molecules that can damage cellular components, including lipids, proteins, and DNA. Persistent oxidative stress can lead to chronic cellular damage, mutations, and an environment that supports cancer development.

4. Inflammation:

- **Chronic Inflammation:** Exposure to harmful chemicals can trigger inflammatory responses. Chronic inflammation is a well-known promoter of cancer, as it can lead to DNA damage, promote cellular proliferation, and inhibit apoptosis (programmed cell death). In the prostate, chronic inflammation can create a microenvironment that supports the initiation and progression of cancer.

Evidence from Research Studies

Numerous studies have investigated the link between exposure to harmful chemicals and prostate cancer risk:

UNVEILING THE CAUSES OF PROSTATE CANCER

-**Cadmium**: A study published in *Environmental Health Perspectives* found that occupational exposure to cadmium was associated with an increased risk of prostate cancer. Workers in industries with high cadmium exposure had higher rates of prostate cancer compared to the general population.

- **Pesticides:** Research in the *American Journal of Epidemiology* reported that agricultural workers exposed to certain pesticides had a significantly higher risk of developing prostate cancer. The study highlighted the importance of protective measures and regulations to reduce exposure.

- **Herbicides**: A study in *Cancer Causes & Control* found that exposure to specific herbicides was linked to an increased risk of aggressive prostate cancer. The findings emphasized the need for further investigation into the safety and long-term effects of these chemicals.

- **Industrial Pollutants Research published in** *Occupational and Environmental Medicine* indicated that workers exposed to industrial pollutants had a higher incidence of prostate cancer. The study underscored the importance of industrial hygiene practices and monitoring for reducing cancer risk.

-Agent Orange: A study published in *Cancer* demonstrated that veterans exposed to Agent Orange had a significantly higher risk of developing aggressive prostate cancer compared to non-exposed veterans. The findings highlight the long-term health impacts of exposure to this toxic herbicide.

PREVENTIVE STRATEGIES FOR PROSTATE CANCER

lifestyle factors such as diet, obesity, physical activity, alcohol consumption, smoking, and exposure to harmful chemicals can influence prostate cancer risk through various mechanisms, including inflammation, oxidative stress, hormonal imbalance, DNA damage, and impaired immune function. Adopting a healthy lifestyle that includes a balanced diet, regular exercise, maintaining a healthy weight, limiting alcohol consumption, avoiding smoking, and minimizing exposure to harmful chemicals can help reduce the risk of developing prostate cancer.

Avoid Exposure to Harmful Chemicals:

1. Protective Equipment:

- Workers in industries with high exposure to harmful chemicals should use appropriate personal protective equipment (PPE), such as gloves, masks, and protective clothing, to minimize exposure.

2. Regulations and Policies:

- Governments and regulatory bodies should enforce stringent regulations to limit occupational exposure to harmful chemicals. Regular monitoring and safety protocols can help protect workers.

3. Education and Training:

- Employers should provide education and training to workers about the risks associated with chemical exposure and the importance of using protective measures. Awareness programs can enhance compliance with safety practices.

4. Regular Health Screening:

- Individuals with occupational exposure to harmful chemicals should undergo regular health screenings, including prostate-specific antigen (PSA) tests and digital rectal exams (DRE), to detect any early signs of prostate cancer.

5. Advocacy for Safer Alternatives:
- Encouraging the development and use of safer alternatives to harmful chemicals can reduce overall exposure and health risks. Research into non-toxic or less harmful substitutes can significantly improve workplace safety.

Occupational and environmental exposure to harmful chemicals such as cadmium, pesticides, herbicides, industrial pollutants, and Agent Orange is a significant risk factor for prostate cancer. These chemicals can disrupt hormonal balance, cause DNA damage, induce oxidative stress, and promote chronic inflammation, all of which contribute to carcinogenesis. Implementing protective measures, regulatory policies, and regular health screenings are essential steps in mitigating these risks. By understanding the mechanisms and taking proactive steps, individuals and organizations can reduce the incidence of prostate cancer associated with harmful chemical exposure and promote healthier working environments.

PREVENTIVE STRATEGIES FOR PROSTATE CANCER

Adopting A Healthy Lifestyle

A) Healthy Diet: Adopting a balanced diet rich in fruits, vegetables, whole grains, and lean proteins can help reduce the risk of prostate cancer. Foods high in antioxidants, such as tomatoes, cruciferous vegetables, and berries, may have protective effects against prostate cancer development. Eating a healthy diet is important for lowering the risk of prostate cancer. Here's why:

1. Balanced Diet: Eating a variety of foods from different food groups is called a balanced diet. This means including fruits, vegetables, whole grains (like brown rice and whole wheat bread), and lean proteins (such as chicken, fish, and beans) in your meals.

2. Fruits and Vegetables: These foods are packed with vitamins, minerals, and antioxidants that help keep your body healthy and protect it from diseases like cancer. Some fruits and veggies, like tomatoes, broccoli, cauliflower, and berries, have special compounds that may specifically help prevent prostate cancer.

5. Antioxidants: Antioxidants are special compounds found in many fruits and vegetables that help protect your cells from damage. This damage can lead to diseases like cancer. Eating a variety of colorful fruits and veggies ensures you get a good mix of antioxidants in your diet Antioxidants are like superheroes that fight off harmful molecules called free radicals, which can damage your cells and increase the risk of cancer. Examples of good fruits and veggies include tomatoes, broccoli, cauliflower, carrots, berries, and citrus fruits like oranges and grapefruits.

3. Whole Grains: Whole grains are a great source of fiber, which helps keep your digestive system working well and may also lower your risk of cancer. Choose whole grain options foods like whole wheat bread, brown rice, oats, and quinoa are rich in fiber and nutrients. Fiber helps keep your digestive system running smoothly and may also help lower the risk of cancer.

4.Lean Proteins: Lean proteins are important for building and repairing tissues in your body. Foods like chicken, turkey, fish, and beans are good sources of protein without a lot of unhealthy fats. Choose lean sources of protein like chicken, turkey, fish, beans, and tofu. These foods provide important nutrients without adding extra saturated fats, which can be harmful to your health.

5) Tomatoes: Tomatoes contain a powerful antioxidant called lycopene, which gives them their red color. Some studies suggest that lycopene may help reduce the risk of prostate cancer. Cooking tomatoes can actually increase the amount of lycopene your body absorbs, so don't be afraid to enjoy them in sauces, soups, and stews.

6) Cruciferous Vegetables: Vegetables like broccoli, cauliflower, Brussels sprouts, and kale are members of the cruciferous family and are rich in compounds called glucosinolates. These compounds may have anti-cancer effects and could help protect against prostate cancer.

By including plenty of fruits, vegetables, whole grains, and lean proteins in your diet, you can give your body the nutrients it needs to stay healthy and lower your risk of prostate cancer. Remember to eat a variety of foods and enjoy meals that are colorful and flavorful!

2. Regular Exercise: Engaging in regular physical activity not only promotes overall health and well-being but may also lower the risk of prostate cancer. Aim for at least 30 minutes of moderate to vigorous exercise most days of the week to reap the benefits of physical activity.

Types of Exercise and Recommendations
To maximize the benefits of physical activity for prostate cancer prevention, aim for at least 30 minutes of moderate to vigorous exercise most days of the week. Here are some effective types of exercise:

1. Aerobic Exercise:
   - Examples: Brisk walking, jogging, swimming, cycling, and dancing.
   - Benefits: Improves cardiovascular health, aids in weight management, and boosts overall stamina.

2. Strength Training:

- Examples: Weight lifting, resistance band exercises, and body-weight exercises like push-ups and squats.

- Benefits: Builds muscle mass, increases metabolism, and enhances bone density.

3. Flexibility and Balance Exercises:

- Examples: Yoga, Pilates, and stretching routines.

- Benefits: Improves flexibility, reduces the risk of injuries, and enhances overall physical balance and coordination.

4. High-Intensity Interval Training (HIIT):

- Examples: Short bursts of intense exercise followed by rest or low-intensity exercise, such as sprinting followed by walking.

- Benefits: Efficient calorie burning, improved cardiovascular fitness, and enhanced metabolic rate.

Practical Tips for Incorporating Exercise

1. **Set Realistic Goals:** Start with achievable goals and gradually increase the intensity and duration of your workouts.

2. **Find Enjoyable Activities:** Choose exercises you enjoy to make it easier to stick with your routine.

3. **Stay Consistent:** Aim to exercise regularly, making it a part of your daily or weekly schedule.

4. **Mix It Up:** Incorporate a variety of exercises to keep your routine interesting and work different muscle groups.

5. **Listen to Your Body:** Pay attention to how your body feels and avoid overexertion. Rest when needed.

6. Find a Workout Buddy:

- Exercising with a friend or family member can provide motivation and make the activity more enjoyable

Engaging in regular physical activity is a powerful tool for maintaining overall health and reducing the risk of prostate cancer. By aiming for at least 30 minutes of moderate to vigorous exercise most days of the week, you can reap numerous health benefits, from weight management and hormone regulation to reduced inflammation and improved immune function. Making exercise a consistent part of your lifestyle not only lowers your risk of prostate cancer but also enhances your quality of life.

How Regular Exercise Lowers Prostate Cancer Risk

Regular exercise is vital for maintaining overall health and well-being, and it can also play a crucial role in lowering the risk of prostate cancer. Here's an in-depth look at how regular physical activity contributes to prostate cancer prevention and the broader benefits it offers:

1. Weight Management:

Exercise helps control weight by burning calories and building muscle. This can prevent weight gain and reduce body fat. Maintaining a healthy weight is important because obesity is linked to an increased risk of aggressive prostate cancer. Fat tissue produces hormones and inflammatory substances that can promote cancer growth. By keeping weight in check, exercise reduces these risk factors.

<u>Impact</u>: Maintaining a healthy weight through exercise can significantly lower the risk of developing prostate cancer.

2. Hormone Regulation:

Physical activity helps balance hormone levels in the body like insulin and insulin-like growth factor 1 (IGF-1). High levels of insulin and insulin-like growth factor (IGF-1) are associated with cancer growth.

<u>Impact</u>: Regular exercise can lower these hormone levels. By keeping these hormone levels in check, exercise can reduce the likelihood of prostate cancer cell development and proliferation

3. Reduced Inflammation:

Regular exercise reduces chronic inflammation in the body. Chronic inflammation can damage cells and lead to cancer. Chronic inflammation is a known risk factor for many types of cancer, including prostate cancer. Exercise has anti-inflammatory effects, helping to reduce inflammation throughout the body. This reduction in inflammation can lower the risk of cellular changes that lead to cancer.

<u>Impact</u>: Lower inflammation levels contribute to a lower risk of prostate cancer and other chronic diseases

4. Improved Immune Function:

Exercise boosts the immune system, enhancing its ability to detect and destroy abnormal cells, including cancer cells

<u>Impact</u>: A stronger immune system is more effective at preventing cancer cells from growing and spreading.

5. Antioxidant Production:

Physical activity increases the production of antioxidants in the body. These antioxidants protect cells by neutralizing free radicals, which are unstable molecules that can cause cellular damage and lead to cancer.

<u>Impact</u>: Higher levels of antioxidants help maintain healthy cells and reduce the risk of prostate cancer. By reducing oxidative stress, exercise helps protect cells from damage.

6. Enhanced Circulation:

- Better blood flow from regular exercise improves the delivery of oxygen and nutrients to cells while removing waste products. This promotes overall cellular health and reduces the risk of cancerous changes.

- <u>Mechanism</u>: Exercise improves blood flow, ensuring that oxygen and nutrients are efficiently delivered to cells while waste products are removed.

- <u>Impact</u>: Better circulation supports overall cellular health and reduces the likelihood of cancerous changes.

PREVENTIVE STRATEGIES FOR PROSTATE CANCER

Types of Exercise for Prostate Cancer Prevention

1. Aerobic Exercise:

- Activities such as brisk walking, jogging, swimming, and cycling improve cardiovascular health and help maintain a healthy weight. Aim for at least 30 minutes of moderate to vigorous aerobic exercise most days of the week.

2. Strength Training:

- Resistance exercises like weightlifting, push-ups, and squats build muscle and improve metabolism. Strength training exercises should be incorporated at least two days a week.

3. Flexibility and Balance Exercises:

- Activities such as yoga and stretching improve flexibility and balance, reducing the risk of injury and promoting overall well-being.

Additional Benefits of Regular Exercise

1. Mental Health:

- Regular physical activity can reduce symptoms of depression and anxiety, improve mood, and enhance overall mental health.

2. Bone Health:

- Weight-bearing exercises strengthen bones, reducing the risk of osteoporosis and fractures.

3. Heart Health:

- Exercise lowers blood pressure, improves cholesterol levels, and reduces the risk of heart disease, which is beneficial for overall longevity.

4. Diabetes Prevention:

- Regular physical activity improves insulin sensitivity, reducing the risk of type 2 diabetes, which is another risk factor for cancer.. Regular exercise is a powerful tool in promoting overall health and reducing the risk of prostate cancer. By incorporating at least 30 minutes of moderate to vigorous physical activity into most days of the week, you can enjoy the numerous benefits of exercise, including better weight management, hormone regulation, reduced inflammation, improved immune function, and enhanced mental well-being. Making exercise a consistent part of your lifestyle is an effective and proactive way to protect your health and lower your risk of prostate cancer.

C. Maintain a Healthy Weight: Obesity and excess body fat have been associated with an increased risk of prostate cancer and disease progression. Maintaining a healthy weight through a balanced diet and regular exercise can help mitigate this risk.

Maintaining a Healthy Weight: An Essential Strategy for Reducing Prostate Cancer Risk

Maintaining a healthy weight is crucial for overall health and well-being, and it plays a significant role in reducing the risk of prostate cancer and its progression. Obesity and excess body fat are associated with numerous health problems, including an increased risk of aggressive prostate cancer. Here's an in-depth look at why maintaining a healthy weight is important and how to achieve it through balanced nutrition and regular physical activity

How Obesity and Excess Body Fat Increase Prostate Cancer Risk

1. Hormonal Imbalance:

Excess body fat, particularly around the abdomen, can lead to hormonal imbalances. Fat tissue produces and stores hormones, including estrogen. Estrogen is a hormone that can influence the development and growth of certain cancers, including prostate cancer. High levels of certain hormones, such as insulin and insulin-like growth factor (IGF-1), associated with obesity, can promote the growth and spread of prostate cancer cells.

2. Chronic Inflammation:

- Obesity often leads to chronic low-grade inflammation in the body. This inflammation can create an environment that supports cancer development and progression. Fat cells release inflammatory substances called cytokines, which can create an environment conducive to cancer development and progression. Inflammatory cells release chemicals that can damage DNA and promote tumor growth.That's Chronic inflammation can damage DNA and promote tumor growth.

3. Insulin Resistance:

- Obesity is a major risk factor for insulin resistance and type 2 diabetes. Insulin resistance results in higher levels of insulin in the blood, which has been linked to an increased risk of prostate cancer.

4. Immune System Dysfunction:

- Excess body fat can impair the immune system's ability to detect and destroy cancer cells. This weakened immune response can allow cancer cells to grow and spread more easily.

Immune System Suppression:

- Excess body fat can impair the immune system's function, reducing its ability to detect and destroy cancerous cells. A weakened immune system allows cancer cells to grow and spread more easily.

4. Metabolic Syndrome:

- Obesity is often associated with metabolic syndrome, a cluster of conditions including high blood pressure, high blood sugar, excess body fat around the waist, and abnormal cholesterol levels. Metabolic syndrome increases the risk of prostate cancer and other chronic diseases.

Benefits of Maintaining a Healthy Weight

1. Reduced Cancer Risk:

- Maintaining a healthy weight helps balance hormone levels, reduce inflammation, and improve insulin sensitivity, all of which contribute to lowering the risk of prostate cancer.

2. Improved Prognosis:
- For men diagnosed with prostate cancer, maintaining a healthy weight can improve outcomes and reduce the risk of disease progression and recurrence.

PREVENTIVE STRATEGIES FOR PROSTATE CANCER

3. Overall Health Improvement:
- A healthy weight is associated with reduced risks of other chronic diseases such as heart disease, diabetes, and

hypertension. It also improves energy levels, mobility, and quality of life.

Strategies for Achieving and Maintaining a Healthy Weight

1. Balanced Diet:

- <u>Eat Plenty of Fruits and Vegetables:</u> These foods are low in calories and high in vitamins, minerals, fiber and antioxidants that help protect against cancer. Aim to fill half your plate with fruits and vegetables at each meal.

<u>Choose Whole Grains:</u> Whole grains like brown rice, whole wheat bread, oats, and quinoa provide more fiber and nutrients than refined grains. They help you feel full longer, which can prevent overeating.

- **Include Lean Proteins:** Incorporate lean sources of protein such as chicken, turkey, fish, beans, and tofu. These foods provide essential nutrients without the added fats found in red and processed meats. Hence, limit red meat and avoid processed meats.

- **Healthy Fats:** Include healthy fats in your diet, such as those found in avocados, nuts, seeds, and olive oil. Avoid trans fats and limit saturated fats.

- **Control Portion Sizes:** Be mindful of portion sizes to avoid overeating. Use smaller plates and listen to your body's hunger and fullness cues.

Limit Sugary Foods and Beverages: Reduce your intake of sugary snacks, desserts, and sugary drinks. These add extra calories with little nutritional value.

- **Control Portion Sizes:** Be mindful of portion sizes to avoid overeating. Use smaller plates and bowls to help control portions, and listen to your body's hunger and fullness cues.

2. Regular Exercise:

- **Aerobic Activities:** Engage in at least 150 minutes of moderate-intensity aerobic exercise (such as brisk walking, cycling, or swimming) or 75 minutes of vigorous-intensity aerobic exercise (such as running or high-intensity interval training) each week.

- **Strength Training:** Include strength training exercises at least two days a week. Activities like weightlifting, resistance band exercises, and body-weight exercises (such as push-ups and squats) help build muscle and boost metabolism.

- **Stay Active Throughout the Day:** Incorporate more physical activity into your daily routine. Take the stairs instead of the elevator, park farther away from your destination, and take short walks during breaks.

3. Healthy Lifestyle Habits:

 - **Stay Hydrated:** Drink plenty of water throughout the day. Sometimes thirst can be mistaken for hunger, leading to overeating.

 - **Get Enough Sleep:** Aim for 7-9 hours of quality sleep each night. Poor sleep can disrupt hormones that regulate hunger and appetite, contributing to weight gain.

 - **Manage Stress:** Chronic stress can lead to emotional eating and weight gain. Practice stress-reducing activities such as yoga, meditation, deep breathing exercises, and spending time in nature.

Behavioral Strategies:

- <u>Set Realistic Goals:</u> Set achievable and specific goals for weight loss and physical activity. Start with small, achievable goals and gradually increase your efforts. Track your progress and celebrate small victories

☐ <u>Stay Consistent</u>: Consistency is key to maintaining a healthy weight. Make healthy eating and regular exercise a part of your daily routine rather than a temporary solution.

☐ <u>Seek Support</u>: Enlist the support of friends, family, or a healthcare professional to help you stay motivated and accountable. Joining a weight loss group or working with a dietitian or personal trainer can also be beneficial.

☐ <u>Manage Stress:</u> High stress levels can lead to overeating and weight gain. Practice stress management techniques such as mindfulness, meditation, deep breathing exercises, and spending time doing activities you enjoy.

- ☐ <u>Keep a Food Diary:</u> Tracking what you eat can help you stay mindful of your food choices and identify areas for improvement.

- ☐ <u>Regular Health Check-Ups:</u> Monitor Your Health, Regular check-ups with your healthcare provider can help you keep track of your weight and overall health. They can provide guidance and support for maintaining a healthy weight and reducing your risk of prostate cancer.

Maintaining a healthy weight is a powerful way to reduce the risk of prostate cancer and improve overall health. By adopting a balanced diet rich in fruits, vegetables, whole grains, and lean proteins, and by engaging in regular physical activity, you can achieve and maintain a healthy weight. This not only lowers your risk of prostate cancer but also enhances your quality of life and reduces the risk of other chronic diseases. Make healthy lifestyle choices a priority to protect your health and well-being for years to come.

4. Limit Alcohol Consumption: Excessive alcohol consumption has been linked to an increased risk of several cancers, including prostate cancer. Limiting alcohol intake to moderate levels (no more than two drinks per day for men) can help reduce this risk.

Limiting Alcohol Consumption as a Preventive Measure for Prostate Cancer: Prostate cancer is a significant health concern for men worldwide, with various lifestyle and genetic factors contributing to its development. One of the controllable lifestyle factors that can influence the risk of prostate cancer is alcohol consumption. Limiting alcohol intake has been shown to reduce the risk of developing various cancers, including prostate cancer. This section explores the relationship between alcohol consumption and prostate cancer, the mechanisms by which alcohol influences cancer risk, and the preventive benefits of moderating alcohol intake.

The Relationship Between Alcohol Consumption and Prostate Cancer

Epidemiological studies have consistently demonstrated a link between alcohol consumption and an increased risk of various cancers, including prostate cancer. Although the exact relationship can be complex and influenced by factors such as the amount and type of alcohol consumed, evidence suggests that heavy and chronic alcohol consumption is particularly harmful.

A meta-analysis published in *Cancer Causes & Control* reviewed numerous studies and found that heavy alcohol consumption (defined as more than two drinks per day) was associated with a higher risk of prostate cancer. Moderate alcohol consumption (up to two drinks per day) showed a less clear association, with some studies indicating a slight increase in risk and others suggesting no significant impact.

Mechanisms by Which Alcohol Increases Prostate Cancer Risk

1. Carcinogenic Compounds and Genotoxicity

- **Metabolism of Ethanol:** Alcohol (ethanol) itself is not a carcinogen, but it is metabolized in the liver to acetaldehyde, a toxic compound and probable human carcinogen. Acetaldehyde can damage DNA and proteins and also interfere with DNA repair, leading to mutations and cellular dysfunction that increase cancer risk.

- **Formation of Reactive Oxygen Species (ROS):** The metabolism of alcohol generates ROS, which can cause oxidative stress. Oxidative stress leads to cellular damage, inflammation, and genetic mutations, all of which contribute to cancer development.

2. Hormonal Imbalance:

- Alteration in Hormone Levels: Alcohol consumption can affect the endocrine system, leading to alterations in hormone levels. In particular, alcohol can increase estrogen levels and potentially decrease testosterone levels. Hormonal imbalances can stimulate the growth of hormone-sensitive tissues, including the prostate, thereby increasing cancer risk.

-Impact on Androgen Receptors: Changes in hormone levels can affect androgen receptors, which play a critical role in the development and progression of prostate cancer. Abnormal activation of these receptors can lead to uncontrolled cell proliferation in the prostate.

PREVENTIVE STRATEGIES FOR PROSTATE CANCER

3. Nutritional Deficiencies:

- Impact on Nutrient Absorption: Chronic alcohol consumption can lead to deficiencies in essential nutrients such as vitamins and minerals, including folate, vitamin B6, and zinc. These nutrients play crucial roles in DNA synthesis and repair as well as cell protection. Lower levels of these nutrients can weaken the body's ability to repair damaged DNA, thus increasing cancer risk.

- Immune System Suppression: Alcohol can impair the immune system, making it less effective at identifying and destroying cancer cells. A weakened immune response allows cancerous cells to proliferate more easily.

4. Behavioral and Lifestyle Factors:

- Poor Diet: Heavy alcohol consumption is often associated with poor dietary choices, such as a diet high in processed foods and low in fruits and vegetables. A poor diet can exacerbate the risk of developing cancer by providing fewer antioxidants and essential nutrients needed for cellular repair and protection.

-Physical Inactivity: Alcohol consumption can contribute to a sedentary lifestyle, which is a known risk factor for prostate cancer. Regular physical activity is important for maintaining a healthy weight and hormonal balance, both of which are protective against cancer.

Benefits of Limiting Alcohol Consumption

1. Reduced Carcinogenic Exposure:

- By limiting alcohol intake, individuals reduce their exposure to acetaldehyde and other carcinogenic byproducts of alcohol metabolism. This lowers the risk of DNA damage and subsequent cancer development.

2. Improved Hormonal Balance:

- Moderating alcohol consumption helps maintain more stable hormone levels. This is particularly important for preventing hormonal imbalances that can promote prostate cancer growth.

3. Enhanced Nutrient Absorption:

- Reducing alcohol intake improves the absorption and utilization of essential nutrients. Adequate levels of vitamins and minerals such as folate, vitamin B6, and zinc are vital for DNA repair and cellular health, reducing the risk of cancer.

4. Stronger Immune Function:

- Limiting alcohol consumption helps preserve immune system function, enabling the body to more effectively detect and eliminate cancer cells. A robust immune system is a critical defense against the development and progression of cancer.

5. Healthier Lifestyle Choices:

- Individuals who limit alcohol consumption are more likely to engage in other healthy behaviors, such as maintaining a balanced diet, exercising regularly, and avoiding tobacco use. These lifestyle factors collectively contribute to a lower risk of prostate cancer.

PREVENTIVE STRATEGIES FOR PROSTATE CANCER

Practical Recommendations for Limiting Alcohol Consumption

1. Set Realistic Limits:

- Aim to consume no more than two alcoholic drinks per day for men. This moderate consumption level is less likely to pose significant health risks.

2. Choose Low-Alcohol Alternatives:

- Opt for beverages with lower alcohol content, such as light beer or wine, instead of high-alcohol spirits.

3. Incorporate Alcohol-Free Days:

- Plan several alcohol-free days each week to give the body time to recover and reduce overall intake.

4. Monitor Drinking Habits:

- Keep a record of alcohol consumption to stay aware of drinking patterns and make adjustments as needed.

5. Seek Support:

- If reducing alcohol intake is challenging, consider seeking support from healthcare professionals, support groups, or counseling services. They can provide strategies and encouragement to help manage and reduce alcohol consumption.

Limiting alcohol consumption is a vital preventive measure for reducing the risk of prostate cancer. By understanding the mechanisms through which alcohol contributes to cancer development and adopting practical strategies to moderate intake, individuals can significantly lower their risk. Combined with other healthy lifestyle choices, reducing alcohol consumption can enhance overall well-being and protect against prostate cancer.

Guidelines and Recommendation for Alcohol Consumption

Given the potential risks associated with alcohol consumption, it is important to adopt responsible drinking habits to mitigate cancer risk. For prostate cancer and other health concerns, the following guidelines are recommended:

Moderation is Key:

Given the potential risks associated with excessive alcohol consumption, it is essential to approach alcohol intake with moderation. For men, this generally means limiting consumption to no more than two drinks per day. <u>A standard drink in the United States typically contains about 14 grams of pure alcohol, equivalent to:</u>
- 12 ounces of beer (5% alcohol content)
- 5 ounces of wine (12% alcohol content)
- 1.5 ounces of distilled spirits (40% alcohol content)

<u>Benefits of Reducing Alcohol Intake:</u>

Reducing alcohol consumption to moderate levels can provide several health benefits, including:

1. Lower Cancer Risk: Limiting alcohol intake reduces the risk of alcohol-related cancers, including prostate cancer.

2. Improved Liver Health: Excessive alcohol consumption is a leading cause of liver disease, including cirrhosis and liver cancer. Moderate drinking helps protect liver function.

3. Cardiovascular Health: While moderate alcohol consumption has been associated with certain cardiovascular benefits, excessive drinking is a risk factor for hypertension, heart disease, and stroke. Moderation helps maintain cardiovascular health.

4. Better Weight Management: Alcohol is calorie-dense and can contribute to weight gain. Reducing intake can help in managing weight, which is an important factor in overall cancer risk reduction.

5. Enhanced Mental Health: Excessive drinking can negatively impact mental health, leading to depression, anxiety, and other issues. Moderate consumption supports better mental well-being.

PREVENTIVE STRATEGIES FOR PROSTATE CANCER

Strategies for Moderating Alcohol Intake:

For those who drink, several strategies can help maintain alcohol consumption at moderate levels:

1. Set Limits: Establish personal limits on how much and how often to drink. Stick to these limits to avoid excessive consumption.

2. Alternate with Non-Alcoholic Drinks: Alternating alcoholic drinks with water or other non-alcoholic beverages can help pace drinking and reduce overall intake.

3. Choose Lower-Alcohol Options: Opt for beverages with lower alcohol content, such as light beer or wine spritzers.

4. Eat While Drinking: Consuming food while drinking slows the absorption of alcohol and can reduce its effects.

5. Plan Alcohol-Free Days: Designate certain days of the week as alcohol-free to ensure that drinking does not become a daily habit.

<u>Understanding the link between excessive alcohol consumption and prostate cancer risk is crucial for making informed lifestyle choices.</u> By limiting alcohol intake to moderate levels, men can significantly reduce their risk of various cancers, including prostate cancer. Embracing moderation not only supports cancer prevention but also contributes to overall health and well-being. Making conscious decisions about alcohol consumption is a proactive step towards a healthier, longer life.

5. Regular Screening: Early detection remains the cornerstone of prostate cancer management. Men should discuss the benefits and risks of prostate cancer screening with their healthcare provider and consider undergoing regular PSA (prostate-specific antigen) testing and digital rectal exams starting at age 50, or earlier for those at higher risk.

Regular Screenings is a preventive measure for Prostate Cancer. Prostate cancer is one of the most common cancers among men, but early detection through regular screenings can significantly improve outcomes and save lives. Screening tests can help identify prostate cancer in its early stages, often before symptoms appear, when the disease is more treatable. Here's an in-depth look at the importance of regular screenings for prostate cancer, the types of screenings available, and practical guidance on when and how to get screened.

Importance of Regular Screenings

1. Early Detection:

- Early detection of prostate cancer increases the chances of successful treatment. Prostate cancer that is caught early is more likely to be confined to the prostate gland, making it easier to treat and cure.

2. Better Prognosis:

- Men diagnosed with early-stage prostate cancer have a higher likelihood of survival and a better quality of life. Early treatment can prevent the cancer from spreading to other parts of the body.

3. Informed Decision-Making:

- Regular screenings provide valuable information that helps men and their healthcare providers make informed decisions about their health. Knowing whether you have prostate cancer can guide treatment choices and management strategies.

4. Risk Management:

- Screenings can identify men at higher risk for developing prostate cancer, allowing for closer monitoring and preventive measures. Men with elevated prostate-specific antigen (PSA) levels or abnormal digital rectal exam (DRE) results can benefit from more frequent follow-up.

PREVENTIVE STRATEGIES FOR PROSTATE CANCER

Types of Prostate Cancer Screenings

1. Prostate-Specific Antigen (PSA) Test:

- The PSA test measures the level of PSA, a protein produced by the prostate gland, in the blood. Elevated PSA levels can indicate prostate cancer, but they can also be caused by other conditions such as benign prostatic hyperplasia (BPH) or prostatitis.

- PSA testing is a simple blood test and is often the first step in prostate cancer screening. Men with high PSA levels may need further testing to confirm the presence of cancer.

2. Digital Rectal Exam (DRE):

- During a DRE, a healthcare provider inserts a gloved, lubricated finger into the rectum to feel the size, shape, and texture of the prostate gland. Abnormalities such as lumps or hard areas can suggest the presence of prostate cancer.

- While DRE is less sensitive than PSA testing, it can detect cancers in men with normal PSA levels and provides additional information about the prostate.

3. Biopsy:

- If PSA and DRE results suggest the possibility of prostate cancer, a biopsy may be performed. During a biopsy, small samples of prostate tissue are taken and examined under a microscope to confirm the presence of cancer cells.

- Biopsies provide definitive evidence of prostate cancer and help determine the aggressiveness of the disease through Gleason scoring

4. Advanced Imaging:

- In some cases, advanced imaging techniques such as MRI or transrectal ultrasound (TRUS) may be used to get a clearer view of the prostate and guide biopsies. These methods can help detect tumors that are not easily found through PSA and DRE alone.

When and How Often to Get Screened

1. General Guidelines:

- The decision to start screening should be based on individual risk factors and discussions with a healthcare provider. Generally, men should consider starting screenings at age 50.

- Men at higher risk, such as African-American men and those with a family history of prostate cancer, should consider starting screenings earlier, around age 40-45.

2. Frequency of Screenings:

- Men with normal PSA levels and DRE results may be advised to repeat screenings every 1-2 years.

- Men with elevated PSA levels or other risk factors may need more frequent monitoring and follow-up tests.

3. Shared Decision-Making:

- It's important for men to engage in shared decision-making with their healthcare providers. This process involves discussing the potential benefits and risks of screenings, considering personal values and preferences, and making informed choices together.

Benefits and Limitations of Screenings

1. Benefits:

- **Improved Survival Rates:** Early detection through screening can lead to earlier treatment and improved survival rates.

- **Reduced Mortality**: Regular screenings have been shown to reduce the mortality rate from prostate cancer.

- **Peace of Mind:** Regular screenings can provide peace of mind for men, knowing they are taking proactive steps to monitor their health.

2. Limitations:

- **False Positives**: PSA tests can sometimes produce false-positive results, leading to unnecessary anxiety and additional testing.

- **Overdiagnosis**: Screenings may detect slow-growing cancers that may never cause symptoms or require treatment, leading to potential overtreatment.

- **Side Effects:** Follow-up procedures, such as biopsies, can have side effects, including pain, bleeding, and infection.

Practical Tips for Prostate Cancer Screenings

1. Know Your Risk:

- Understand your personal risk factors, such as age, race, family history, and lifestyle, and discuss them with your healthcare provider.

2. Stay Informed:

- Keep up-to-date with the latest guidelines and recommendations for prostate cancer screenings from reputable health organizations.

PREVENTIVE STRATEGIES FOR PROSTATE CANCER

3. Schedule Regular Check-Ups:

- Regular check-ups with your healthcare provider can ensure timely screenings and prompt follow-up if abnormalities are found.

4. Communicate Openly:

- Discuss any symptoms, concerns, or changes in your health with your healthcare provider. Open communication can lead to earlier detection and better outcomes.

Regular screenings are a crucial preventive measure for prostate cancer. By detecting the disease early, screenings can significantly improve survival rates and quality of life. Men should engage in informed discussions with their healthcare providers to determine the best screening schedule based on their individual risk factors. Regular check-ups, staying informed, and maintaining open communication with healthcare providers are key steps in proactively managing prostate health and reducing the risk of prostate cancer.

Conclusion of Chapter Two

While the exact causes of prostate cancer are still being elucidated, understanding the various risk factors and adopting preventive strategies can help reduce the likelihood of developing this disease. By making informed lifestyle choices, maintaining regular health screenings, and staying vigilant about potential symptoms, individuals can take proactive steps towards prostate cancer prevention and overall health promotion.

CHAPTER 3: Do I Have Prostate Cancer? Screening and Detection

CHAPTER OUTLINE

SCREENING AND DETECTION.

Understanding Prostate Cancer

Risk Factors for Prostate Cancer:

Screening Methods for Prostate Cancer

- Prostate-Specific Antigen (PSA) Test

- ☐ Digital Rectal Exam (DRE)
- ☐ Advanced Screening Methods
    - ☐ MRI and Ultrasound
    - ☐ Biomarker Test

Procedure for confirming the diagnosis

- Prostate Biopsy
- Imaging to confirm the extent of the cancer using bone scan, and CT scan
- Genetic Testing
- Role and Importance of regular screening

Balancing the Benefits and risk of screening.

Recommendations for Prostate Cancer Screening.

Prostate cancer, a leading cause of cancer in men, is often asymptomatic in its early stages, making regular screening and early detection vital. This chapter provides an in-depth exploration of the methods used to detect prostate cancer, the interpretation of results, and the importance of understanding personal risk factors. It aims to educate readers on the intricacies of prostate cancer screening, empowering them to make informed decisions about their health.

Understanding Prostate Cancer

Prostate cancer originates in the prostate gland, a small, walnut-shaped gland in men that produces seminal fluid. The cancer can grow slowly and remain confined to the gland, or it can be more aggressive and spread to other parts of the body. Understanding whether one has prostate cancer typically involves several steps: recognizing risk factors, undergoing screening tests, and, if necessary, confirming the diagnosis with further medical evaluations.

MALE REPRODUCTIVE SYSTEM

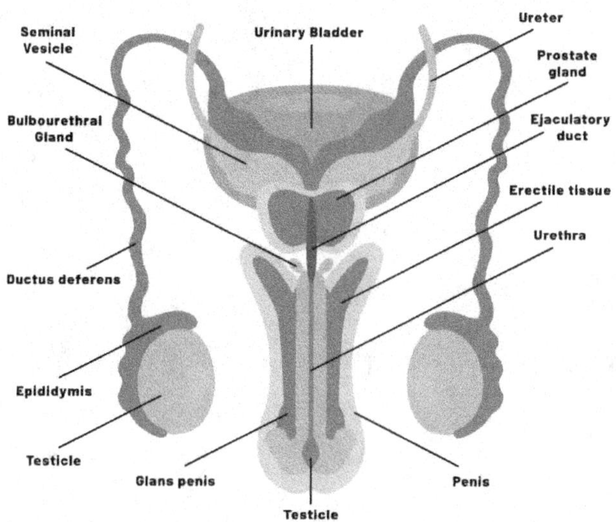

Prostate Cancer

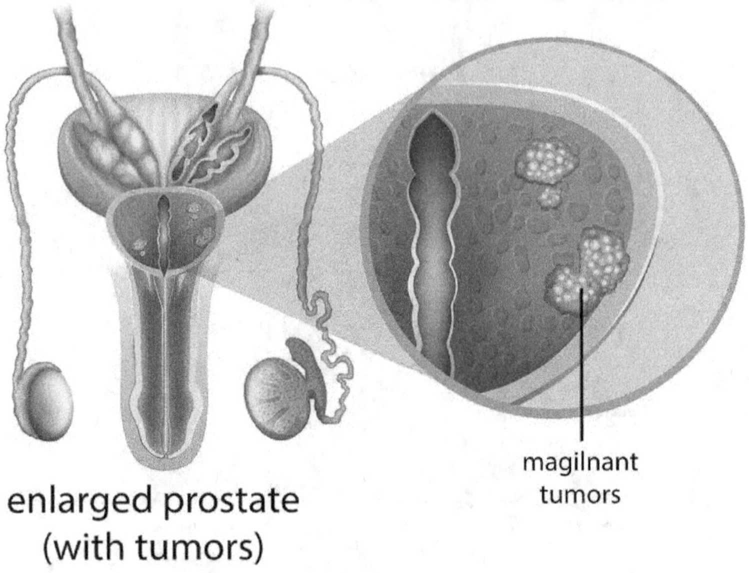

enlarged prostate
(with tumors)

Just a quick reminder about Risk Factors for Prostate Cancer:

1. Age:

- Age is the most significant risk factor for prostate cancer. The risk increases exponentially after the age of 50. Most cases are diagnosed in men over 65.

2. Family History:

- Having a father, brother, or other close relatives with prostate cancer significantly increases the risk. Genetic factors can play a crucial role in predisposing men to the disease.

3. Race and Ethnicity:

- African American men have a higher risk of developing prostate cancer compared to men of other races. They are also more likely to be diagnosed at an advanced stage and have a higher mortality rate.

4. Genetic Mutations:

- Mutations in genes such as BRCA1, BRCA2, and others involved in DNA repair can increase the risk of prostate cancer. Men with these genetic mutations should consider earlier and more frequent screening.

5. Lifestyle Factors:

- Diet, obesity, and exposure to certain chemicals can influence prostate cancer risk. High-fat diets and obesity have been linked to an increased risk, while regular physical activity may reduce it.

Screening Methods for Prostate Cancer

1. Prostate-Specific Antigen (PSA) Test:

- What is PSA?

- PSA is a protein produced by the prostate gland. Elevated levels of PSA in the blood can be an early indicator of prostate cancer, though benign conditions like prostatitis and benign prostatic hyperplasia (BPH) can also raise PSA levels.

- How is the Test Conducted?

- The PSA test involves drawing a blood sample and measuring the PSA level in the blood. Results are typically reported in nanograms per milliliter (ng/mL).

- Interpreting PSA Results:

- PSA levels below 4.0 ng/mL are generally considered normal, but this can vary with age. Levels between 4.0 and 10.0 ng/mL are considered borderline and may require further testing. Levels above 10.0 ng/mL are more suggestive of prostate cancer and warrant additional investigation.

2. Digital Rectal Exam (DRE):

- What is DRE?

- During a DRE, a healthcare provider inserts a gloved, lubricated finger into the rectum to feel the prostate gland. This exam can detect abnormalities such as lumps or hard areas that might indicate cancer.

- How is the Exam Conducted?

- The patient typically bends forward at the waist or lies on their side with knees drawn to the chest. The provider gently examines the prostate through the rectal wall.

- Interpreting DRE Results:

- A normal DRE result means the prostate feels smooth and of normal size. Any irregularities, such as lumps or hardness, may require further testing.

3. Advanced Screening Methods:

<u>- MRI and Ultrasound:</u>

- Multiparametric MRI (mpMRI) can provide detailed images of the prostate and help identify suspicious areas. Ultrasound, often used in conjunction with a biopsy, helps guide the procedure to ensure accuracy.

- Biomarker Tests:

- Newer tests that measure specific biomarkers in the blood, urine, or tissue can provide additional information about prostate cancer risk and aggressiveness. Examples include the Prostate Health Index (PHI) and the 4Kscore test.

Confirming the Diagnosis

1. Prostate Biopsy:

- What is a Biopsy?

- A prostate biopsy involves taking small samples of prostate tissue to examine under a microscope for cancer cells. This is typically done using a needle guided by ultrasound.

- How is it Conducted?

- The procedure can be done through the rectum (transrectal biopsy) or the perineum (transperineal biopsy). Local anesthesia is used to minimize discomfort.

- Interpreting Biopsy Results:

- The tissue samples are examined for cancer cells, and the results are graded using the Gleason score, which helps determine the aggressiveness of the cancer. Scores range from 6 (less aggressive) to 10 (most aggressive).

2. Additional Tests:

- Imaging

- If cancer is confirmed, additional imaging tests such as bone scans, CT scans, or PET scans may be conducted to determine if the cancer has spread beyond the prostate.

Screening Methods for Prostate Cancer

- **Genetic Testing**

- Genetic tests can identify specific mutations that may influence treatment decisions and provide information about familial risk.

The Role of Regular Screening

1. <u>Early Detection and Treatment:</u>

- Regular screening allows for the detection of prostate cancer at an early stage, when treatment options are more effective and less invasive. Early-stage cancer confined to the prostate gland can often be treated successfully with surgery, radiation, or other therapies.

2. <u>Monitoring High-Risk Individuals:</u>

- For men with a higher risk of prostate cancer due to genetic factors, family history, or other risk factors, regular screening is essential. It allows for close monitoring and timely intervention if cancer develops.

3. <u>Informed Decision-Making:</u>

- Regular screening provides critical information that helps men make informed decisions about their health. Understanding the benefits and risks of screening, along with personal risk factors, allows for personalized healthcare strategies.

Balancing the Benefits and Risks of Screening

1. **Overdiagnosis and Overtreatment:**

- One of the challenges of prostate cancer screening is the potential for overdiagnosis—identifying cancers that may never cause symptoms or health problems. This can lead to overtreatment, with side effects from interventions that may not have been necessary.

2. **Personalized Screening Strategies:**

- Screening guidelines should be tailored to individual risk profiles. Men at average risk may start screening at age 50, while those at higher risk should consider beginning earlier. Discussions with healthcare providers about the frequency and type of screening tests are crucial.

3. **Shared Decision-Making:**

- Shared decision-making between patients and healthcare providers is essential. Men should be fully informed about the potential outcomes of screening and treatment options, enabling them to make choices aligned with their values and preferences.

Practical Recommendations for Prostate Cancer Screening

1. <u>Start Discussions Early</u>:

- Men should begin discussing prostate cancer screening with their healthcare providers at age 50, or earlier if they have risk factors such as family history or genetic predispositions.

2. <u>Understand the Tests</u>:

- Familiarize yourself with the PSA test and DRE, including what the tests involve, how results are interpreted, and the implications of abnormal findings.

3. <u>Consider Advanced Screening Methods</u>:

- For those with elevated PSA levels or abnormal DRE results, consider additional tests like MRI or biomarker tests to provide more detailed information.

4. <u>Stay Informed:</u>

- Keep up with the latest research and guidelines on prostate cancer screening. New developments in testing and treatment can influence screening strategies.

5. <u>Maintain Regular Check-Ups:</u>

- Regular health check-ups and screenings are essential for early detection. Even if initial tests are normal, ongoing monitoring is important, especially for those at higher risk.

Prostate cancer screening is a critical component of men's health, providing a pathway to early detection and effective management of the disease. By understanding the risk factors, the screening methods available, and the importance of regular monitoring, men can take proactive steps to protect their health. Engaging in informed discussions with healthcare providers, considering personal risk factors, and staying up-to-date with screening recommendations are essential strategies for reducing the burden of prostate cancer. Through vigilant screening and early intervention, the prospects for successful treatment and long-term survival are greatly enhanced. Me

CHAPTER 4: DIAGNOSIS AND STAGING

CHAPTER OUTLINE

DIAGNOSIS AND STAGING

DIAGNOSIS

A. Screening Test

<u>Prostate-Specific Antigen (PSA) Test</u>

- ☐ The Science Behinds PSA
- ☐ Methodology of the PSA Test
- ☐ Interpreting PSA Levels
- ☐ Factors Affecting PSA Levels
    - ☐ Benign Prostatic Hyperplasia (BPH)
    - ☐ Prostatitis
    - ☐ Prostate Cancer
    - ☐ Other Influences
- ☐ Benefits of PSA Testing
- ☐ Limitations and Controversies

- Recent Advances and Future Directions

Digital Rectal Exam

- What is a Digital Rectal Exam (DRE)
- The Procedure of a DRE
- Significance of the DRE
- Benefits of the DRE
- Limitations of the DRE
- When is a DRE recommended
- Practical tips for patients who wants to undergo DRE

B. Advanced Diagnostic Test

Multiparametric MRI (mpMRI).

- What is Multiparametric MRI (mpMRI)
- How mpMRI works
- Benefit of mpMRI
- Limitations of mpMRI

- ☐ Transrectal Biopsy
- ☐ Transperineal Biopsy
- ☐ Pathology Report
- ☐ Importance of Pathology Report

STAGING

Gleason Score

- ☐ What is the Gleason Score
- ☐ Gleason Score Ranges
- ☐ How is the Gleason Score determind
- ☐ Primary and Secondary grades
- ☐ Combining Grades to form the Gleason Score
- ☐ Reporting the Gleason Score
- ☐ Importance of the Gleason Score

Staging of Prostate cancer, TNM

- ☐ T(Tumor)
- ☐ N (Nodes)
- ☐ M(Metastasis)

Importance of Accurate Staging

Additional staging tools

- ☐ Bone Scan
- ☐ CT Scan
- ☐ PET Scan

Staging groups

- ☐ Stage I: Characteristics, Description & Treatments
- ☐ Stage II: Characteristics, Description & Treatments
- ☐ Sage III: Characteristics, Description & Treatments
- ☐ Stage IV: Characteristics, Description & Treatments

Risk Stratification

- ☐ Low Risk Prostate Cancer: Description and Management
- ☐ Intermediate Risk Prostate Cancer: Description and Management
- ☐ High Risk Prostate Cancer: Description and Management

Diagnostic Pathways and Follow-Up

- ☐ Initial Evaluation
- ☐ Confirming the Diagnosis
- ☐ Ongoing Monitoring
- ☐ Multidisciplinary Approach

Patients Involvement and Decision Making

- ☐ Informed Consent
- ☐ Patient Education
- ☐ Shared Decision-Making

Prostate cancer diagnosis and staging are critical steps in determining the extent of the disease and planning appropriate treatment. This chapter delves into the processes and tools used to diagnose prostate cancer, interpret the results, and stage the cancer. Understanding the intricacies of how prostate cancer is diagnosed and staged is crucial for making informed decisions about treatment and management.

Diagnosis of Prostate Cancer

The diagnosis of prostate cancer typically follows a series of tests and evaluations, starting with screening tests like PSA and DRE, followed by more definitive diagnostic procedures.

1. Screening Tests

Prostate-Specific Antigen (PSA) Test: Elevated levels of PSA in the blood can indicate the presence of prostate cancer, although benign conditions like prostatitis and benign prostatic hyperplasia (BPH) can also raise PSA levels.

Prostate-Specific Antigen (PSA) Test: Comprehensive Overview

The Prostate-Specific Antigen (PSA) test is a critical tool in the early detection and management of prostate cancer. This test measures the level of PSA, a protein produced by the prostate gland, in the blood. Elevated levels can indicate the presence of prostate cancer, though benign conditions like prostatitis and benign prostatic hyperplasia (BPH) can also raise PSA levels. To provide a more detailed understanding, let's delve into various aspects of the PSA test, including its scientific basis, methodology, interpretation, benefits, limitations, and recent advancements.

The Science Behind PSA

PSA is a glycoprotein enzyme produced by both normal and malignant cells of the prostate gland. It plays a role in liquefying semen, which is crucial for sperm motility. In healthy individuals, most PSA is released into the semen, with only a small amount entering the bloodstream. However, disruptions to the prostate's architecture, such as those caused by cancer, inflammation, or other conditions, can increase the leakage of PSA into the blood.

Methodology of the PSA Test

1. Sample Collection:

- A simple blood sample is collected from a vein in the arm, typically taking only a few minutes. This sample is then sent to a laboratory for analysis.

2. Laboratory Analysis:

- The blood sample is analyzed using immunoassays, which are techniques that use antibodies to detect and measure specific proteins like PSA. These tests can be very sensitive, detecting even small amounts of PSA.

Interpreting PSA Levels

1. <u>Normal vs. Elevated Levels:</u>

- Traditionally, a PSA level of 4.0 ng/mL or lower is considered normal for most men, although levels can vary based on age, race, and other factors.

- Levels above 4.0 ng/mL are typically considered elevated and may warrant further investigation.

2. Age-Specific Ranges:

- PSA levels tend to increase with age. Age-specific reference ranges can help improve the specificity of the test. For example, a PSA level of 2.5 ng/mL might be considered elevated for a man in his 40s, but normal for someone in his 70s.

3. PSA Velocity:

- The rate of increase in PSA levels over time, known as PSA velocity, can also be an important indicator. A rapid increase in PSA levels may suggest the presence of aggressive prostate cancer.

4. PSA Density:

- PSA density considers the PSA level in relation to the volume of the prostate. This can be measured using ultrasound. Higher PSA density may indicate a higher likelihood of prostate cancer.

5. <u>Free vs. Bound PSA:</u>

- PSA exists in two main forms in the blood: free (not bound to proteins) and bound (attached to blood proteins). The ratio of free to total PSA can help differentiate between prostate cancer and benign conditions. Lower ratios of free PSA are more indicative of prostate cancer.

Factors Affecting PSA Levels

1. <u>Benign Prostatic Hyperplasia (BPH):</u>

- BPH is a non-cancerous enlargement of the prostate that commonly occurs with aging. It can raise PSA levels and cause urinary symptoms, complicating the interpretation of PSA test results.

2. <u>Prostatitis:</u>

- Inflammation or infection of the prostate gland can significantly elevate PSA levels. Symptoms may include pelvic pain, difficulty urinating, and fever.

3. <u>Prostate Cancer:</u>

- Elevated PSA levels can indicate prostate cancer, especially if levels are significantly above the normal range or rising quickly. However, further testing is required to confirm the presence of cancer.

4. <u>Other Influences:</u>

- Activities like ejaculation, vigorous exercise (e.g., cycling), and medical procedures involving the prostate (e.g., DRE, biopsy) can temporarily elevate PSA levels. Men are advised to avoid these activities before a PSA test.

Benefits of PSA Testing

1. <u>Early Detection:</u>

- The PSA test can detect prostate cancer at an early stage when it is more likely to be confined to the prostate and more treatable.

2. <u>Monitoring:</u>

- For men diagnosed with prostate cancer, PSA tests are essential for monitoring the disease's progression and the effectiveness of treatments.

3. <u>Risk Stratification:</u>

- PSA levels, along with other factors, help stratify men into different risk categories, guiding decisions about further testing and treatment options.

Limitations and Controversies

1. <u>False Positives:</u>

- Elevated PSA levels can be caused by benign conditions, leading to unnecessary anxiety, further testing, and invasive procedures.

2. <u>Overdiagnosis and Overtreatment:</u>

- PSA testing can identify slow-growing cancers that may never cause symptoms or become life-threatening. Treating these cancers can expose men to side effects without significant benefits.

3. <u>Variable Interpretation:</u>

- PSA levels can fluctuate due to various factors, making it challenging to interpret a single test result. Repeated testing and considering trends over time are often necessary.

4. <u>Balancing Benefits and Risks:</u>

- The decision to undergo PSA screening should be based on a thorough discussion with a healthcare provider, considering individual risk factors and personal preferences.

Recent Advances and Future Directions

1. Refinement of PSA Testing:

- New approaches to PSA testing, such as measuring PSA isoforms and molecular markers, aim to improve the test's specificity and reduce false positives.

2. Genomic Testing:

- Advances in genomic testing are helping to identify genetic mutations and molecular profiles associated with prostate cancer, offering more personalized screening and treatment strategies.

3. Imaging Techniques:

- Improved imaging techniques, such as multiparametric MRI, can provide more detailed information about the prostate and help guide biopsies, improving the accuracy of prostate cancer diagnosis.

4. Liquid Biopsies:

- Research into liquid biopsies, which analyze cancer-related DNA and other markers in the blood, holds promise for non-invasive cancer detection and monitoring.

☐ The PSA test remains a cornerstone of prostate cancer screening, offering the potential for early detection and improved outcomes. However, its limitations necessitate careful consideration and personalized decision-making. Men should discuss their individual risk factors, the benefits and risks of PSA testing, and the potential for further testing with their healthcare providers. By staying informed about the latest advancements and screening guidelines, men can make educated decisions about their prostate health and screening practices.

Digital Rectal Exam (DRE):
A physical examination where a healthcare provider feels the prostate through the rectal wall to detect abnormalities.

Digital Rectal Exam (DRE): A Comprehensive Guide

The Digital Rectal Exam (DRE) is a crucial procedure in the early detection and diagnosis of prostate abnormalities, including cancer. This physical examination allows healthcare providers to palpate the prostate gland through the rectal wall to identify any irregularities in size, shape, or texture. Understanding the DRE, its procedure, significance, benefits, and limitations is essential for men's health awareness and proactive management of prostate conditions.

What is a Digital Rectal Exam (DRE)?

A Digital Rectal Exam (DRE) is a clinical procedure performed by a healthcare provider to examine the prostate gland and other lower pelvic organs. The term "digital" refers to the use of a finger (digitus in Latin), not digital technology. During the exam, the provider inserts a lubricated, gloved finger into the rectum to feel the prostate gland through the rectal wall.

The Procedure of a DRE

1. Preparation:

- The patient is usually asked to undress from the waist down and may be provided with a gown. The patient can lie on their side with knees drawn to the chest, bend over the examination table, or lie on their back with feet in stirrups. The position depends on the patient's comfort and the provider's preference.

2. Performing the Exam:

- The healthcare provider puts on a glove and applies lubricant to the index finger.

- The provider then gently inserts the finger into the patient's rectum and palpates the prostate gland. The examination typically lasts a few minutes and may cause slight discomfort but should not be painful.

- The provider feels for the size, shape, and texture of the prostate, checking for any hard areas, lumps, or other abnormalities.

3. Post-Exam Discussion:

- After the exam, the healthcare provider discusses the findings with the patient. If any abnormalities are detected, further tests may be recommended, such as a PSA test, ultrasound, or biopsy.

Significance of the DRE

1. <u>Early Detection of Prostate Cancer:</u>

- The DRE can detect prostate abnormalities that may indicate cancer, especially in cases where PSA levels are not significantly elevated. Early detection is crucial for effective treatment and better outcomes.

2. Assessment of Prostate Size and Shape:

- The DRE allows the provider to assess the overall size and shape of the prostate. An enlarged prostate can indicate benign prostatic hyperplasia (BPH), a common condition in older men that can cause urinary symptoms.

3. Detection of Other Conditions:

- Apart from prostate cancer and BPH, the DRE can help identify other conditions such as prostatitis (inflammation of the prostate), rectal tumors, and anal fissures.

Benefits of the DRE

1. Non-Invasive and Quick:

- The DRE is a non-invasive procedure that can be completed in a few minutes during a routine physical examination. It requires no special equipment or preparation.

2. Immediate Results:

- The healthcare provider can immediately share findings with the patient, allowing for prompt discussion of next steps if any abnormalities are detected.

3. Complementary to PSA Testing:

- The DRE is often used in conjunction with the PSA test to improve the accuracy of prostate cancer screening. While the PSA test measures a protein level in the blood, the DRE provides a physical assessment of the prostate.

Limitations of the DRE

1. <u>Subjective Nature:</u>

   - The effectiveness of the DRE depends on the skill and experience of the healthcare provider. Interpretation can be subjective, and small or deep-seated tumors may be missed.

2. <u>Limited Reach:</u>

   - The DRE can only assess the posterior and lateral aspects of the prostate. Tumors located in the anterior part of the prostate may not be detectable through a DRE.

3. <u>Patient Discomfort:</u>

   - Some patients may experience discomfort or anxiety about the procedure. Clear communication and reassurance from the provider can help alleviate these concerns.

When is a DRE Recommended?

1. Routine Screening:

   - Many healthcare providers recommend routine DREs for men over the age of 50 as part of regular health check-ups. Men at higher risk for prostate cancer, such as those with a family history of the disease or of African-American descent, may be advised to start screening earlier.

2. Symptomatic Patients:

   - Men experiencing symptoms such as difficulty urinating, frequent urination, pain during urination, or lower back pain may undergo a DRE to help diagnose the underlying cause.

3. Follow-Up Assessments:

- For men diagnosed with prostate conditions, periodic DREs may be used to monitor the progress of the disease and the effectiveness of treatments.

Practical Tips for Patients

1. Discuss Concerns:

- Patients should feel comfortable discussing any concerns or questions with their healthcare provider before the exam. Understanding the procedure can help reduce anxiety.

2. Relax During the Exam:

- Relaxing the muscles can help minimize discomfort during the DRE. Deep breathing techniques can be helpful.

3. Follow Post-Exam Recommendations:

- If the provider recommends further tests or follow-up appointments based on the DRE findings, it's important to follow through to ensure any potential issues are promptly addressed.

□ The Digital Rectal Exam (DRE) is a vital tool in the early detection and management of prostate abnormalities, including cancer. Despite its limitations, the DRE provides valuable information about the prostate's size, shape, and texture, which can help identify conditions such as prostate cancer, BPH, and prostatitis. When used in conjunction with PSA testing, the DRE enhances the accuracy of prostate cancer screening and helps guide further diagnostic and treatment decisions. Open communication with healthcare providers, understanding the procedure, and regular screenings are key components of effective prostate health management.

2. Advanced Diagnostic Tests

- Multiparametric MRI (mpMRI): This imaging test provides detailed pictures of the prostate and helps identify suspicious areas that may need further investigation. It combines anatomical imaging with functional imaging, offering a comprehensive view of the prostate.

Advanced Diagnostic Tests: Multiparametric MRI (mpMRI)

Multiparametric MRI (mpMRI) represents a significant advancement in prostate cancer diagnostics. This sophisticated imaging technique provides detailed and comprehensive pictures of the prostate, aiding in the identification of suspicious areas that may require further investigation. By combining various imaging modalities, mpMRI enhances the accuracy and effectiveness of prostate cancer detection, characterization, and staging.

What is Multiparametric MRI (mpMRI)?

Multiparametric MRI (mpMRI) is an advanced form of magnetic resonance imaging (MRI) specifically tailored to evaluate the prostate gland. Unlike standard MRI, mpMRI integrates multiple imaging sequences to provide a detailed and multifaceted view of the prostate. These sequences include:

1. T2-Weighted Imaging (T2WI):

- This sequence provides high-resolution anatomical images of the prostate, highlighting the different zones of the gland and any structural abnormalities.

2. Diffusion-Weighted Imaging (DWI):

- DWI measures the movement of water molecules within tissues. Cancerous tissues often restrict water diffusion, making them appear differently from normal tissues. This sequence is crucial for detecting and characterizing prostate lesions.

3. Dynamic Contrast-Enhanced Imaging (DCE):

- DCE involves the injection of a contrast agent into the bloodstream, followed by rapid imaging to track the contrast as it moves through the prostate. This sequence assesses blood flow patterns, which can help identify areas with increased vascularity often associated with tumors.

4. Magnetic Resonance Spectroscopy (MRS):

- MRS analyzes the chemical composition of prostate tissues, measuring concentrations of specific metabolites. It can provide additional information about the biochemical environment of the prostate, though it is less commonly used than the other sequences.

How mpMRI Works

1. Preparation:

- Before the scan, patients may be asked to follow specific dietary restrictions and instructions to empty the bowels. This helps minimize artifacts and improves image quality.

2. During the Scan:

- The patient lies on an MRI table, which slides into the MRI machine. The procedure typically lasts between 30 to 60 minutes.

- The patient must remain still to ensure clear images. In some cases, a rectal coil may be used to enhance image resolution, although this is becoming less common with advances in external coils.

3. Imaging Sequences:

- The MRI machine captures images using the different sequences (T2WI, DWI, DCE, and optionally MRS). These images are then combined and analyzed to provide a comprehensive view of the prostate.

Benefits of mpMRI

1. Enhanced Detection:

- mpMRI improves the detection of clinically significant prostate cancers, particularly those located in areas difficult to assess with traditional methods. It is especially useful for identifying tumors in the anterior part of the prostate.

2. Guidance for Biopsies:

- By pinpointing suspicious areas, mpMRI can guide targeted biopsies, increasing the likelihood of detecting significant cancers while reducing the number of unnecessary biopsies.

3. Accurate Staging:

- mpMRI provides detailed images that help determine the extent of cancer within and beyond the prostate gland, aiding in accurate staging and treatment planning.

4. Risk Stratification:

- The technique helps differentiate between aggressive and indolent cancers, assisting clinicians in risk stratification and decision-making regarding treatment options.

5. Non-Invasive:

- mpMRI is a non-invasive procedure with no radiation exposure, making it a safer alternative to other diagnostic methods like CT scans or PET scans.

Limitations of mpMRI

1. Accessibility and Cost:

- mpMRI is more expensive and less widely available than standard imaging techniques. Access may be limited in some regions or healthcare systems.

2. Interpretation Variability:

- The accuracy of mpMRI depends on the expertise of the radiologist interpreting the images. Variability in interpretation can affect diagnostic accuracy.

3. Patient Factors:

- Certain factors, such as the presence of metal implants, severe claustrophobia, or inability to remain still, can limit the use of mpMRI or affect image quality.

4. False Positives and Negatives:

- While mpMRI is highly sensitive, it can still produce false positives (identifying benign areas as suspicious) and false negatives (missing some cancerous areas), necessitating correlation with clinical findings and other tests.

Clinical Applications of mpMRI

1. Initial Diagnosis:

- mpMRI is used to evaluate men with elevated PSA levels or abnormal findings on a digital rectal exam (DRE). It helps identify regions of the prostate that may need a biopsy.

2. Active Surveillance:

- For men on active surveillance for low-risk prostate cancer, mpMRI can monitor for disease progression, potentially reducing the need for repeated biopsies.

3. Pre-Biopsy Evaluation:

- mpMRI can be performed before a biopsy to guide targeted biopsies, improving the likelihood of detecting clinically significant cancer.

4. Post-Treatment Monitoring:

- After treatments such as surgery or radiation therapy, mpMRI can monitor for signs of recurrence, providing valuable information for ongoing management.

Advancements and Future Directions

1. Standardization of Reporting:

- The development of standardized reporting systems, such as the Prostate Imaging Reporting and Data System (PI-RADS), has improved the consistency and accuracy of mpMRI interpretations.

2. Integration with Other Technologies:

- Combining mpMRI with other diagnostic technologies, such as genetic testing and molecular biomarkers, holds promise for more precise and personalized prostate cancer management.

3. Artificial Intelligence (AI):

- AI and machine learning are being integrated into mpMRI analysis to enhance image interpretation, reduce variability, and improve diagnostic accuracy.

4. Patient-Specific Models:

- Advances in imaging technology and computational modeling are paving the way for creating patient-specific models of the prostate, enhancing individualized treatment planning.

Multiparametric MRI (mpMRI) is a powerful diagnostic tool that provides comprehensive imaging of the prostate, aiding in the detection, characterization, and staging of prostate cancer. By combining anatomical and functional imaging, mpMRI offers detailed insights that surpass traditional imaging techniques. Despite its limitations, the benefits of mpMRI in improving diagnostic accuracy, guiding targeted biopsies, and aiding in treatment planning are substantial. As technology advances and accessibility improves, mpMRI is poised to play an increasingly vital role in the early detection and management of prostate cancer.

- **Biomarker Tests:** These tests measure specific proteins or genetic material in blood, urine, or tissue samples to help assess the risk of prostate cancer. Examples include the Prostate Health Index (PHI) and the 4Kscore test.

Biomarker Tests for Prostate Cancer: A Comprehensive Overview

Biomarker tests are an integral part of modern prostate cancer diagnostics, providing valuable information about the presence, risk, and progression of the disease. These tests measure specific proteins, genetic material, or other molecular markers in blood, urine, or tissue samples, helping to refine the assessment of prostate cancer risk and guide clinical decision-making. Two prominent examples of biomarker tests are the Prostate Health Index (PHI) and the 4Kscore test. Here, we will explore these tests in detail, discussing their mechanisms, applications, benefits, and limitations.

What are Biomarker Tests?

Biomarker tests detect and measure biological molecules that indicate the presence or risk of disease. In the context of prostate cancer, these biomarkers can include proteins produced by the prostate gland, genetic alterations, and other molecular signals associated with cancerous changes.

Key Biomarker Tests for Prostate Cancer

1. Prostate Health Index (PHI):

  - <u>Description:</u>

   - The Prostate Health Index (PHI) is a blood test that combines three different PSA measurements: total PSA, free PSA, and [-2]proPSA. These values are integrated into a mathematical formula to produce the PHI score.

  - <u>Mechanism:</u>

   - Total PSA measures the overall level of prostate-specific antigen in the blood.

- Free PSA refers to the portion of PSA that is not bound to proteins in the blood. Lower ratios of free PSA to total PSA are associated with a higher risk of prostate cancer.

- [-2]proPSA is a specific subform of free PSA that is more closely associated with prostate cancer.

- <u>Application:</u>

- PHI is used to improve the accuracy of prostate cancer detection in men with elevated PSA levels. It helps differentiate between prostate cancer and benign conditions such as benign prostatic hyperplasia (BPH).

- <u>Benefits:</u>

- PHI enhances the specificity of prostate cancer screening, reducing unnecessary biopsies.

- It provides a more nuanced risk assessment compared to total PSA alone.

-<u>Limitations:</u>

- While PHI improves diagnostic accuracy, it is not definitive and must be used in conjunction with other clinical information.

2. 4Kscore Test:

- <u>Description:</u>

- The 4Kscore test is a blood test that measures four kallikrein protein levels: total PSA, free PSA, intact PSA, and human kallikrein 2 (hK2). These measurements are combined with clinical information to estimate the risk of high-grade prostate cancer (Gleason score ≥7).

- <u>Mechanism:</u>

- Total PSA and free PSA levels provide a baseline understanding of PSA dynamics.

- Intact PSA is a precursor form of PSA that remains bound to proteins.

- Human kallikrein 2 (hK2) is another protein closely related to PSA, involved in prostate cancer biology.

- <u>Application:</u>

- The 4Kscore test is used to assess the likelihood of high-grade prostate cancer in men with abnormal PSA levels or digital rectal exam (DRE) findings. It aids in decision-making regarding the need for a biopsy.

- <u>Benefits:</u>

- The test provides a comprehensive risk assessment, helping to identify men at higher risk for aggressive prostate cancer.

- It helps reduce unnecessary biopsies and associated complications.

- <u>Limitations:</u>

- Like PHI, the 4Kscore test is not definitive and should be interpreted alongside other clinical data.

Benefits of Biomarker Tests.

1. Enhanced Diagnostic Accuracy:

- Biomarker tests provide a more precise risk assessment for prostate cancer, improving the specificity of screening programs and reducing the rate of false positives.

2. Personalized Risk Assessment:

- By incorporating multiple biomarkers and clinical factors, these tests offer personalized insights into an individual's risk of prostate cancer, aiding in tailored decision-making.

3. Reduction of Unnecessary Biopsies:

- By distinguishing between high-risk and low-risk cases, biomarker tests help avoid unnecessary biopsies and their potential side effects, such as pain, bleeding, and infection.

4. Monitoring and Management:

- Biomarker tests can be used to monitor disease progression in men with known prostate cancer or those under active surveillance, providing ongoing risk assessment and guiding treatment decisions.

Limitations of Biomarker Tests

1. Cost and Accessibility:

- Biomarker tests can be more expensive than traditional PSA testing and may not be covered by all insurance plans, potentially limiting access for some patients.

2. Interpretation Variability:

- The interpretation of biomarker test results requires expertise and should be done by healthcare providers experienced in prostate cancer management.

3. Not Standalone Tests:

- Biomarker tests should not be used in isolation. They are most effective when used in conjunction with other diagnostic tools, such as PSA tests, DRE, and imaging studies.

Future Directions in Biomarker Testing
1. Integration with Genomic Testing:

- Advances in genomic testing are identifying new biomarkers that can further refine prostate cancer risk assessment and personalized treatment strategies.

2. Development of New Biomarkers:

- Research continues to identify and validate new biomarkers that could improve the sensitivity and specificity of prostate cancer screening and diagnosis.

3. Improved Risk Stratification Models:
   - Combining biomarker tests with advanced statistical and computational models can enhance risk stratification and clinical decision-making.

Biomarker tests, such as the Prostate Health Index (PHI) and the 4Kscore test, represent significant advancements in prostate cancer diagnostics. These tests offer more accurate and personalized risk assessments, improving early detection and reducing unnecessary interventions. While they have limitations, their integration into clinical practice, alongside traditional methods and emerging technologies, holds promise for more effective prostate cancer management.

Patients should discuss the potential benefits and limitations of biomarker tests with their healthcare providers to make informed decisions about their prostate health.

3. Prostate Biopsy

- Procedure: A biopsy involves taking small samples of prostate tissue to examine under a microscope for cancer cells. It is usually guided by transrectal ultrasound (TRUS) or MRI.

- **Types of Biopsy:**

- **Transrectal Biopsy**: A needle is inserted through the rectum to obtain tissue samples.

- **Transperineal Biopsy:** A needle is inserted through the skin between the scrotum and rectum, often used when transrectal biopsy is not possible.

- **Pathology Report:** The biopsy samples are analyzed to determine the presence of cancer cells, their grade, and other characteristics. The pathology report provides crucial information for staging and treatment planning.

Prostate Biopsy: Comprehensive Overview

Prostate biopsy is a critical diagnostic procedure used to detect the presence of prostate cancer. It involves taking small tissue samples from the prostate gland, which are then examined under a microscope to identify cancer cells. The procedure is typically guided by imaging techniques such as transrectal ultrasound (TRUS) or magnetic resonance imaging (MRI) to ensure accuracy. Understanding the biopsy procedure, its types, and the resulting pathology report is essential for patients and healthcare providers to make informed decisions about prostate cancer diagnosis and treatment.

Procedure

A prostate biopsy is performed to collect tissue samples from the prostate gland for microscopic examination. This procedure is usually recommended when other tests, such as the Prostate-Specific Antigen (PSA) test or Digital Rectal Exam (DRE), indicate a potential abnormality that warrants further investigation.

1. Preparation:

 - Prior to the biopsy, patients may be advised to stop certain medications that can increase bleeding risk, such as blood thinners.

- An enema may be administered to clear the rectum, and antibiotics are often prescribed to prevent infection.

2. Anesthesia:

- Local anesthesia is typically used to numb the area around the prostate, ensuring that the patient is comfortable during the procedure.

3. Imaging Guidance:

- The biopsy is guided by imaging techniques to accurately target the prostate and identify suspicious areas.

- **Transrectal Ultrasound (TRUS)**: This involves inserting an ultrasound probe into the rectum to visualize the prostate and guide the biopsy needle.

- **MRI**: In some cases, MRI is used in conjunction with ultrasound

(MRI/ultrasound fusion) to enhance the accuracy of the biopsy.

4. Sample Collection:

- A biopsy needle is inserted through the rectum or perineum (the skin between the scrotum and rectum) to collect tissue samples from different areas of the prostate.

- Typically, 10-12 samples are taken to ensure a comprehensive examination of the gland.

5. Post-Procedure Care:

- Patients may experience mild discomfort, blood in the urine, semen, or stool, and should avoid strenuous activities for a few days. Antibiotics continue to be taken as prescribed to prevent infection.

Types of Biopsy

There are two main types of prostate biopsy: transrectal biopsy and transperineal biopsy. The choice between these methods depends on various factors, including patient anatomy, previous biopsy results, and specific clinical considerations.

1. Transrectal Biopsy:

- Procedure:

- During a transrectal biopsy, an ultrasound probe is inserted into the rectum to visualize the prostate. A biopsy needle is then guided through the rectal wall to obtain tissue samples.

- Advantages:

- It is the most commonly performed type of prostate biopsy due to its accessibility and the ability to use TRUS for real-time imaging.

- Disadvantages:

- This method carries a higher risk of infection because the needle passes through the rectal wall, which contains bacteria.

2. Transperineal Biopsy:

- **Procedure**:

- In a transperineal biopsy, the biopsy needle is inserted through the perineum. This approach is often used when transrectal biopsy is not feasible or when a more comprehensive sampling is needed.

- Advantages:

- It has a lower risk of infection compared to transrectal biopsy since the needle does not pass through the rectal wall.

- It allows for better access to certain areas of the prostate, including the anterior regions.

- Disadvantages:

- This method may require general or spinal anesthesia and can be more complex and time-consuming.

Pathology Report

The pathology report is a detailed document that provides the results of the prostate biopsy. It is crucial for diagnosing prostate cancer and planning appropriate treatment. The report typically includes several key elements:

1. Cancer Presence:

- The pathologist examines the biopsy samples under a microscope to determine whether cancer cells are present. If cancer is detected, the report will specify the location and extent of the cancer within the samples.

2. Gleason Score:

- The Gleason score is a grading system used to evaluate the aggressiveness of prostate cancer. It is based on the microscopic appearance of the cancer cells.

- The score is composed of two numbers, each ranging from 1 to 5, which represent the most common and second most common patterns of cancer cells in the samples. These two numbers are added together to produce a Gleason score ranging from 6 to 10.

- Gleason scores of 6 indicate low-grade cancer.

- Scores of 7 indicate intermediate-grade cancer.

- Scores of 8 to 10 indicate high-grade, more aggressive cancer.

3. Tumor Volume:

- The report may include information on the tumor volume, indicating the percentage of each biopsy core that contains cancer. This helps assess the extent of the disease.

4. Perineural Invasion:

- The presence of perineural invasion (cancer cells surrounding or tracking along a nerve within the prostate) can be noted, which may have implications for the potential spread of the cancer.

5. Other Findings:

- The report may also describe other relevant findings, such as inflammation, high-grade prostatic intraepithelial neoplasia (PIN), or atypical small acinar proliferation (ASAP), which could suggest a higher risk of cancer.

Importance of the Pathology Report

1. Treatment Planning:

   - The information in the pathology report is essential for staging the cancer and determining the appropriate treatment options. For instance, low-grade cancers may be managed with active surveillance, while high-grade cancers may require more aggressive treatments such as surgery, radiation, or hormonal therapy.

2. Prognostic Information:

   - The Gleason score and other pathological findings provide important prognostic information, helping to predict the likely behavior of the cancer and guide long-term management strategies.

3. Patient Counseling:

   - Detailed pathology reports enable healthcare providers to effectively communicate the diagnosis and treatment options to patients, allowing for informed decision-making and personalized care.

A prostate biopsy is a critical diagnostic procedure for detecting and characterizing prostate cancer. Whether performed via the transrectal or transperineal route, it provides essential tissue samples for microscopic examination. The resulting pathology report offers valuable insights into the presence, grade, and extent of cancer, playing a pivotal role in treatment planning and prognostication. Understanding the biopsy process, its types, and the importance of the pathology report is key to navigating the complex landscape of prostate cancer diagnosis and management. Regular screenings and discussions with healthcare providers about biopsy options and outcomes can significantly impact early detection and successful treatment of prostate cancer.

4. Gleason Score

- What is the Gleason Score?: The Gleason score is a grading system that evaluates the aggressiveness of prostate cancer based on the appearance of cancer cells in the biopsy samples. It ranges from 6 (less aggressive) to 10 (most aggressive).

- How is it Determined?: The pathologist examines the patterns of cancer cells and assigns a primary and secondary grade, which are then added together to form the Gleason score.

Gleason Score: Comprehensive Overview

What is the Gleason Score?

The Gleason score is a critical grading system used to evaluate the aggressiveness of prostate cancer. It is based on the microscopic examination of prostate cancer cells in biopsy samples, assessing how much the cancerous tissue differs from normal prostate tissue. This score helps determine the likely behavior of the cancer and guides treatment decisions. The Gleason score ranges from 6 to 10, with lower scores indicating less aggressive cancer and higher scores indicating more aggressive and potentially more dangerous cancer.

1. Gleason Score Ranges:

- Score 6: Represents low-grade cancer. The cancer cells look more like normal cells and are usually slower-growing.

- Score 7: Represents intermediate-grade cancer. It is divided into:

- 3+4=7: Indicates that the primary pattern is less aggressive, and the secondary pattern is more aggressive.

- 4+3=7: Indicates that the primary pattern is more aggressive, and the secondary pattern is less aggressive.

- Scores 8-10: Represents high-grade cancer. These scores indicate that the cancer cells look very different from normal cells and are more likely to grow and spread quickly.

How is the Gleason Score Determined?

The determination of the Gleason score is a detailed process performed by a pathologist who examines the biopsy samples of prostate tissue under a microscope. The process involves several steps to ensure an accurate assessment:

1. Biopsy Sample Collection

- Multiple tissue samples (cores) are taken from different areas of the prostate during a biopsy. Typically, 10-12 cores are collected to provide a comprehensive overview of the prostate's condition.

2. Microscopic Examination:

- The pathologist examines the samples to identify patterns of cancer cells. Prostate cancer cells tend to form glandular structures, and the degree to which these structures resemble normal prostate glands varies.

3. Pattern Grading:

- The pathologist assigns a grade to the two most predominant patterns of cancer cells observed in the samples. These grades range from 1 to 5:

- **Grade 1:** The cancer cells look very similar to normal prostate cells and form well-defined glands.

- **Grade 2:** The cells are still well-formed but show more variation in size and shape.

- **Grade 3:** The cells are less uniform and the glands are more irregular.

- **Grade 4:** The cells are even more abnormal and form few glandular structures.

- **Grade 5:**The cancer cells do not form glands at all and are highly irregular, resembling sheets or nests of cells.

4. Primary and Secondary Grades:

- The primary grade is assigned to the most common pattern observed in the cancerous tissue.

- The secondary grade is assigned to the second most common pattern.

5. Combining Grades to Form the Gleason Score:

- The primary and secondary grades are added together to form the Gleason score. For example, if the most common pattern is grade 3 and the second most common pattern is grade 4, the Gleason score would be 3+4=7.

6. Reporting the Gleason Score:

- The Gleason score is reported as the sum of the primary and secondary grades, along with the individual grades (e.g., Gleason 3+4=7). This provides a detailed understanding of the cancer's aggressiveness.

Importance of the Gleason Score

1. Risk Stratification:

- The Gleason score is a crucial factor in stratifying patients into different risk categories. It helps identify which patients are at low, intermediate, or high risk of disease progression and metastasis.

2. Treatment Planning:

- The score informs treatment decisions, guiding whether active surveillance, surgery, radiation therapy, or other treatments are appropriate. For instance:

- Low-Grade Cancer (Gleason 6): May be suitable for active surveillance, especially in older men or those with other significant health issues.

- Intermediate-Grade Cancer (Gleason 7): Often requires a **combination of treatments, such as surgery or radiation**, sometimes along with hormonal therapy.

- **High-Grade Cancer** (Gleason 8-10): Typically necessitates more aggressive treatment due to the higher likelihood of spread and recurrence.

3. Prognostic Value:

- The Gleason score provides valuable prognostic information. Higher scores are associated with a poorer prognosis, higher risk of recurrence, and lower survival rates.

4. Guiding Clinical Trials:

- The Gleason score is also used in clinical trials to select appropriate candidates and to stratify patients based on the aggressiveness of their cancer, ensuring that trial results are accurately interpreted.

5. Patient Counseling:

   - Understanding the Gleason score helps healthcare providers explain the nature and severity of the cancer to patients, facilitating informed decision-making and setting realistic expectations about outcomes.

The Gleason score is an essential tool in the diagnosis and management of prostate cancer. By grading the aggressiveness of cancer based on the microscopic appearance of prostate cells, it provides critical insights into the likely behavior of the disease. The process of determining the Gleason score involves a detailed examination of biopsy samples and a careful assessment of cancer cell patterns. This score plays a pivotal role in risk stratification, treatment planning, prognostication, and patient counseling. Understanding the Gleason score helps patients and healthcare providers navigate the complexities of prostate cancer diagnosis and make informed choices about care and management strategies.

Staging of Prostate Cancer

Staging is the process of determining the extent and spread of cancer within the body. Accurate staging is essential for selecting the most appropriate treatment plan.

1. TNM Staging System

- **T (Tumor)**: Describes the size and extent of the primary tumor.

  - **T1:** Tumor is not detectable by DRE or imaging but is found in tissue samples.

  - **T2:** Tumor is confined within the prostate.

  - **T3:** Tumor extends beyond the prostate capsule.

  - **T4:** Tumor has invaded nearby structures other than seminal vesicles.

- **N** (Nodes): Indicates whether the cancer has spread to nearby lymph nodes.

  - **N0**: No regional lymph node involvement.

  - **N1:** Regional lymph nodes are involved.

- **M (Metastasis):** Indicates whether the cancer has spread to distant parts of the body.

  - **M0**: No distant metastasis.

  - **M1:** Distant metastasis is present.

Prostate Cancer Staging: A Comprehensive Overview

Staging is a critical process in the management of prostate cancer, as it determines the extent of the disease within the body. Accurate staging guides treatment decisions, helps predict outcomes, and facilitates communication among healthcare providers. The TNM staging system is the most widely used method for staging prostate cancer, providing detailed information about the tumor's size, lymph node involvement, and the presence of metastasis.

1. TNM Staging System

The TNM staging system is a standardized approach developed by the American Joint Committee on Cancer (AJCC) and the Union for International Cancer Control (UICC). It classifies cancer into three **primary components: Tumor (T), Nodes (N), and Metastasis (M).**

T (Tumor): Describes the size and extent of the primary tumor.

- **T1:**Tumor is not detectable by Digital Rectal Exam (DRE) or imaging but is found in tissue samples.
  - **T1a:** Cancer is found incidentally in less than 5% of the tissue resected (e.g., during surgery for benign prostatic hyperplasia).
  - **T1b**: Cancer is found in more than 5% of the tissue resected.

- **T1c:** Cancer is identified by needle biopsy, typically due to elevated PSA levels.

- **T2**:Tumor is confined within the prostate.

- **T2a**: Cancer involves one-half or less of one side (lobe) of the prostate.

- **T2b**: Cancer involves more than one-half of one lobe but not both lobes.

- **T2c**: Cancer involves both lobes of the prostate.

- **T3**: Tumor extends beyond the prostate capsule.

- **T3a**: Cancer extends beyond the prostate capsule but does not invade the seminal vesicles.

- **T3b**: Cancer has invaded the seminal vesicles.

- **T4**: Tumor has invaded nearby structures other than seminal vesicles (e.g., bladder neck, rectum, pelvic wall).

 - This indicates a more advanced stage of cancer that may require more aggressive treatment.

N (Nodes): Indicates whether the cancer has spread to nearby lymph nodes.

- **N0:** No regional lymph node involvement.

 - This means the cancer has not spread to the lymph nodes near the prostate, suggesting a localized disease.

- **N1**: Regional lymph nodes are involved.

 - This indicates that cancer cells have been found in the lymph nodes close to the prostate, suggesting a higher stage and potentially a more aggressive disease.

M (Metastasis): Indicates whether the cancer has spread to distant parts of the body.

- **M0**: No distant metastasis.

  - This means the cancer has not spread to distant organs or tissues, which is a favorable prognostic sign.

- **M1**: Distant metastasis is present.

  - **M1a**: Cancer has spread to distant lymph nodes.

  - **M1b**: Cancer has spread to bones.

  - **M1c**: Cancer has spread to other distant sites (e.g., lungs, liver).

Importance of Accurate Staging

Accurate staging is essential for several reasons:

1. Treatment Planning:

- Staging helps determine the most appropriate treatment strategy. For example, localized prostate cancer (T1 or T2) might be treated with surgery or radiation, while advanced stages (T3 or T4) might require a combination of treatments, including hormone therapy and chemotherapy.

2. Prognosis:

- The stage of the cancer provides critical information about the likely course and outcome of the disease. Lower stages generally have a better prognosis and higher survival rates compared to higher stages.

3. Clinical Trials:

- Staging allows for the selection of appropriate candidates for clinical trials, ensuring that patients receive experimental treatments that are suitable for their stage of disease.

4. Patient Counseling:

- Knowing the stage of cancer helps healthcare providers give patients a clear understanding of their condition, treatment options, and expected outcomes. This information is crucial for informed decision-making.

5. Monitoring and Follow-up:

- Staging provides a baseline against which to measure the effectiveness of treatment and monitor for potential recurrence. Regular follow-ups and imaging studies are based on the initial stage of the cancer.

Prostate cancer staging is a vital step in the management and treatment of the disease. The TNM staging system provides a detailed framework for understanding the extent of cancer spread, which is crucial for selecting appropriate treatment options, predicting outcomes, and facilitating patient care. Accurate staging helps ensure that patients receive the most effective and personalized care, improving their chances of successful treatment and long-term survival.

2. Additional Staging Tools

- Bone Scan: Detects whether cancer has spread to the bones, which is common in advanced prostate cancer.

- CT Scan: Provides detailed images of the body's internal structures to check for spread to lymph nodes or other organs.

- PET Scan: Uses a radioactive tracer to detect cancer cells throughout the body.

3. Staging Groups

- **Stage I:** Cancer is confined to a small area of the prostate and is not aggressive (Gleason score 6, PSA <10 ng/mL).

- **Stage II:** Cancer is more advanced but still confined to the prostate (Gleason score 6-7, PSA 10-20 ng/mL).

- **Stage III:** Cancer has spread beyond the prostate to nearby tissues (Gleason score 7-8, PSA >20 ng/mL).

- **Stage IV:** Cancer has spread to distant parts of the body (Gleason score 8-10, any PSA level).

Staging Groups of Prostate Cancer: Comprehensive Overview

Prostate cancer staging groups help categorize the extent and aggressiveness of the disease, which is crucial for determining the most appropriate treatment and predicting patient outcomes. The staging groups are based on the combination of the TNM classification, Gleason score, and PSA levels. Understanding these staging groups provides a clear framework for healthcare providers and patients to approach the management of prostate cancer effectively.

Stage I

Characteristics:

- **Tumor Extent (T):** The cancer is confined to a small area of the prostate and is not detectable by a digital rectal exam (DRE) or imaging. It may have been found incidentally during surgery for another condition or identified through a needle biopsy.

- **Gleason Score:** 6 or less, indicating low-grade, less aggressive cancer.

- **PSA Level**: Less than 10 ng/mL, suggesting a lower likelihood of aggressive disease.

Description:

Stage I prostate cancer represents an early stage where the cancer is limited to a very small part of the prostate. The cells appear similar to normal cells and the tumor grows slowly. Due to its limited extent and low aggressiveness, Stage I cancer often has an excellent prognosis and may be managed with active surveillance, particularly in older men or those with significant comorbidities. Treatment options may also include surgery or radiation therapy, depending on the patient's age, health, and preferences.

Stage II

Characteristics:

-Tumor Extent (T): The cancer is more advanced but still confined to the prostate. It can be detected through a DRE or imaging and may be more extensive within the prostate.

- **Gleason Score**: 6-7, indicating a moderate level of aggressiveness.

- **PSA Level**: Between 10 and 20 ng/mL, suggesting a higher risk compared to Stage I.

Description:

Stage II prostate cancer indicates that the tumor is larger and may be found in more than one part of the prostate but has not spread beyond the prostate itself. It is categorized into two sub-stages:

- **Stage IIA**: Cancer is present in one-half or less of one side of the prostate (Gleason 6, PSA 10-20 ng/mL).

- **Stage IIB:** Cancer is present in more than one-half of one side but not both sides, or it involves both sides but still confined to the prostate (Gleason 7, PSA 10-20 ng/mL).

Treatment options for Stage II prostate cancer often include surgery (radical prostatectomy), radiation therapy, and sometimes hormonal therapy. The choice of treatment depends on various factors, including the patient's age, overall health, and personal preferences.

Stage III

Characteristics:

- **Tumor Extent (T):** The cancer has spread beyond the prostate to nearby tissues but has not yet reached distant organs.

- **Gleason Score**: 7-8, indicating a high level of aggressiveness.
- **PSA Level**: Greater than 20 ng/mL, which is associated with a higher risk of spread and recurrence.

Description:

Stage III prostate cancer signifies that the tumor has extended beyond the prostate capsule, potentially invading nearby tissues such as the seminal vesicles but not distant sites. It is categorized into:

- Stage IIIA: Cancer has spread beyond the prostate but has not invaded the seminal vesicles (Gleason 7-8, PSA >20 ng/mL).
- Stage IIIB: Cancer has invaded the seminal vesicles or adjacent structures.

This stage of prostate cancer typically requires more aggressive treatment due to the increased risk of progression. Treatment options may include a combination of surgery, radiation therapy, and hormonal therapy. In some cases, chemotherapy may be considered, especially if there is a high risk of recurrence.

Stage IV

Characteristics:

- **Tumor Extent (T):** The cancer has spread to distant parts of the body, such as bones, lymph nodes, or other organs.
- Gleason Score: 8-10, indicating very high aggressiveness.
- **PSA Level:** Can be any level, as the primary concern is the extent of spread rather than the PSA value alone.

Description:

Stage IV prostate cancer is the most advanced stage, indicating that the cancer has metastasized to distant sites. It is further divided into:

- Stage IVA: Cancer has spread to regional lymph nodes (N1).

- Stage IVB: Cancer has spread to distant lymph nodes, bones, or other organs (M1).

Treatment for Stage IV prostate cancer focuses on controlling the spread of the disease and alleviating symptoms. Options include hormonal therapy to reduce androgen levels, chemotherapy, targeted therapy, immunotherapy, and palliative care to manage symptoms and improve quality of life. Clinical trials may also be an option for some patients, offering access to new and experimental treatments.

Summary note on Staging

Prostate cancer staging groups provide a systematic approach to understanding the extent and aggressiveness of the disease, guiding treatment decisions and prognosis. Stage I indicates a very localized and low-risk cancer, while Stage II represents more extensive but still localized disease. Stage III cancer has begun to spread beyond the prostate, and Stage IV cancer has metastasized to distant parts of the body. Accurate staging is essential for selecting the most appropriate treatment plan, predicting outcomes, and facilitating effective communication between patients and healthcare providers. Understanding these staging groups empowers patients to make informed decisions about their care and management.

Risk Stratification

Risk stratification helps to categorize prostate cancer into different risk levels based on PSA levels, Gleason score, and tumor stage. This classification guides treatment decisions.

1. Low-Risk:

- PSA <10 ng/mL

- Gleason score ≤6

- T1-T2a stage

2. Intermediate-Risk:

- PSA 10-20 ng/mL

- Gleason score 7

- T2b-T2c stage

3. High-Risk:

- PSA >20 ng/mL

- Gleason score 8-10

- T3-T4 stage

Comprehensive Note on Prostate Cancer Risk Stratification

Risk stratification in prostate cancer is a crucial process that helps categorize the disease into different risk levels based on specific clinical parameters. These parameters include PSA levels, Gleason score, and tumor stage. By accurately classifying prostate cancer, healthcare providers can tailor treatment strategies to each patient's individual risk profile, improving outcomes and optimizing care.

 1. Low-Risk Prostate Cancer

Criteria:

- PSA Level: Less than 10 ng/mL

- Gleason Score: 6 or less

- Tumor Stage: T1-T2a

Description:

Low-risk prostate cancer is characterized by a combination of low PSA levels, low Gleason scores, and early-stage tumors. This category indicates that the cancer is confined to the prostate and has a low likelihood of aggressive behavior or rapid progression.

- PSA Level (<10 ng/mL): PSA, or prostate-specific antigen, is a protein produced by both normal and malignant prostate cells. Low PSA levels suggest a smaller tumor burden and lower likelihood of cancer spreading beyond the prostate.
- Gleason Score (≤ 6): The Gleason score assesses the aggressiveness of cancer based on how prostate cancer cells look under a microscope. A score of 6 or less indicates well-differentiated cells that resemble normal cells and are less likely to grow and spread quickly.

- Tumor Stage (T1-T2a): Tumor stage describes the extent of cancer within the prostate. T1 tumors are not palpable or visible by imaging but may be found incidentally. T2a tumors are confined to one-half or less of one lobe of the prostate.

Management:
- Active Surveillance: Monitoring the cancer closely with regular PSA tests, DREs, and periodic biopsies to ensure it does not progress.
- Definitive Treatment: Options may include radical prostatectomy (surgical removal of the prostate) or radiation therapy, particularly for younger patients or those preferring to eliminate the cancer.

2. Intermediate-Risk Prostate Cancer
Criteria:
- PSA Level: 10-20 ng/mL

- Gleason Score: 7
- Tumor Stage: T2b-T2c

Description:

Intermediate-risk prostate cancer indicates a higher potential for progression compared to low-risk cancer. This category includes moderate PSA levels, a moderate Gleason score, and tumors that are still confined to the prostate but may be larger or involve more of the prostate.

- PSA Level (10-20 ng/mL): PSA levels in this range suggest a higher tumor burden than low-risk cancer, indicating a greater chance of the cancer growing or spreading.
- Gleason Score (7): A Gleason score of 7 is considered intermediate. It can be further categorized into 3+4=7, which is less

aggressive, and 4+3=7, which is more aggressive.

- Tumor Stage (T2b-T2c): T2b tumors involve more than one-half of one lobe of the prostate but not both lobes. T2c tumors involve both lobes.

Management:

-Definitive Treatment: Radical prostatectomy or radiation therapy is often recommended. These treatments may be combined with hormone therapy, especially if the Gleason score is 4+3=7, indicating a more aggressive cancer.

- Active Surveillance: In some cases, particularly for older patients or those with other significant health issues, active surveillance may be considered, though less commonly than in low-risk cases.

3. High-Risk Prostate Cancer

Criteria:

- PSA Level: Greater than 20 ng/mL

- Gleason Score: 8-10

- Tumor Stage: T3-T4

Description:

High-risk prostate cancer is characterized by high PSA levels, high Gleason scores, and advanced tumor stages. This category indicates a significant risk of aggressive disease that is more likely to spread beyond the prostate.

-PSA Level (>20 ng/mL): Elevated PSA levels suggest a substantial tumor burden and a higher probability of metastasis.
- Gleason Score (8-10): These scores represent poorly differentiated cancer cells that are likely to grow and spread rapidly. Gleason scores of 8-10 indicate a high degree of malignancy.

-Tumor Stage (T3-T4): T3 tumors extend beyond the prostate capsule, and T4 tumors invade nearby structures such as the bladder neck, rectum, or pelvic wall.

Management:

- Aggressive Treatment: A combination of therapies is often required. This may include radical prostatectomy, radiation therapy, and long-term hormone therapy to reduce androgen levels that fuel cancer growth.

- Chemotherapy: Used in cases where cancer has spread beyond the prostate or is not responding to hormone therapy.

-Clinical Trials: Patients with high-risk prostate cancer may be candidates for clinical trials exploring new treatments or combination therapies.

-Palliative Care: Focused on managing symptoms and maintaining quality of life, particularly for those with advanced disease.

Key Points on Risk stratification

Risk stratification is an essential aspect of managing prostate cancer, enabling personalized treatment plans based on the specific characteristics of the disease. By categorizing prostate cancer into low, intermediate, and high-risk groups, healthcare providers can tailor interventions to each patient's needs, improving outcomes and optimizing care. Understanding these risk levels helps patients make informed decisions about their treatment options and participate actively in their care planning.

Diagnostic Pathways and Follow-Up

1. Initial Evaluation:

- Following elevated PSA or abnormal DRE results, further diagnostic tests such as mpMRI and biopsy are conducted.

- A detailed medical history and physical examination are essential to assess overall health and potential risk factors.

2. Confirming the Diagnosis:

- Biopsy results and imaging studies confirm the presence of prostate cancer and provide detailed information on the cancer's characteristics.

3. Ongoing Monitoring:

- Patients diagnosed with prostate cancer require regular follow-up to monitor disease progression, response to treatment, and manage any side effects.

4. Multidisciplinary Approach:

- Prostate cancer diagnosis and staging benefit from a multidisciplinary team approach, involving urologists, oncologists, radiologists, and pathologists to ensure comprehensive care.

Patient Involvement and Decision-Making

1. Informed Consent:

- Patients should be fully informed about the diagnostic tests, potential outcomes, and implications for treatment. Informed consent involves discussing the risks, benefits, and alternatives to each procedure.

2. Patient Education:

- Understanding the diagnostic process and staging system helps patients actively participate in their care. Educational materials, support groups, and counseling services can provide valuable support.

3. Shared Decision-Making:

- Treatment decisions should be made collaboratively, considering the patient's values, preferences, and overall health. Shared decision-making ensures that patients are comfortable with their care plan and are more likely to adhere to it.

Facts about Diagnosing and Staging.

Diagnosing and staging prostate cancer are complex processes that involve various tests and evaluations. Early and accurate diagnosis, coupled with precise staging, is crucial for determining the most effective treatment strategy. By understanding the diagnostic tools and staging systems, patients can actively participate in their care, making informed decisions that improve their prognosis and quality of life. Regular follow-up and a multidisciplinary approach ensure that patients receive comprehensive and personalized care throughout their cancer journey.

CHAPTER 5: What Are My Options?

Factors Influencing Treatments Decision

- ☐ Stage and grade of the Cancer
- ☐ Patient's Age and Life Expectancy
- ☐ Overall Health and Comorbidities

- ☐ Potential Side Effects and Quality of Life
- ☐ Patient's Preferences

Treat Options

1. Active Surveillance
2. Surgery
3. Radiation
4. Proton Beam Radiation
5. Radiopharmaceuticals
6. Hormone Therapy
7. Chemotherapy
8. Immunotherapy
9. Bisphosphonate Therapy
10. Cryotherapy or Cryosurgery
11. Prostate Cancer Vaccine
12. High-intensity Focused Ultrasound

When faced with a prostate cancer diagnosis, understanding the available treatment options is crucial. This chapter provides a comprehensive overview of the different approaches to managing prostate cancer, from active surveillance to advanced therapies. Each option comes with its benefits, risks, and considerations, and the choice of treatment depends on various factors including the stage and grade of cancer, the patient's overall health, and personal preferences.

Factors Influencing Treatment Decisions for Prostate Cancer

Making informed decisions about prostate cancer treatment involves considering various factors that can significantly impact the choice and outcome of treatment. Here are detailed explanations of the key factors influencing these decisions:

1. Stage and Grade of Cancer

The stage and grade of prostate cancer are pivotal in determining the appropriate treatment strategy.

- Early-Stage Cancer (Localized):

- <u>Description:</u> In early-stage prostate cancer, the cancer is confined to the prostate gland. This stage includes T1 and T2 categories in the TNM system.

 - Treatment Options:

   - <u>Active Surveillance</u>: Suitable for men with low-risk, slow-growing cancer.

   - <u>Surgery (Radical Prostatectomy):</u> Removal of the prostate gland, potentially curing the cancer if it hasn't spread.

   - <u>Radiation Therapy:</u> Using high-energy rays to target and kill cancer cells, available as external beam radiation or brachytherapy (internal radiation).

- Advanced Cancer (Locally Advanced or Metastatic):

- <u>Description</u>: In advanced stages, cancer has spread beyond the prostate to nearby tissues or other parts of the body. This includes T3, T4, N1, and M1 categories.

- <u>Treatment Options:</u>

-<u>Hormone Therapy (Androgen Deprivation Therapy)</u>: Reduces levels of male hormones that can promote cancer growth.

- <u>Chemotherapy</u>: Uses drugs to kill rapidly dividing cancer cells.

-<u>Targeted Therapies and Immunotherapy:</u> Newer treatments that target specific cancer cell mechanisms or boost the body's immune response against cancer.

2. Patient's Age and Life Expectancy

The age and life expectancy of a patient are crucial in choosing an appropriate treatment plan.

- <u>Younger Patients:</u>

  - <u>Description</u>: Generally healthier and with a longer life expectancy, younger patients may benefit from more aggressive treatments aimed at curing the cancer.

  - <u>Treatment Choices:</u>

  - <u>Aggressive Treatments</u>: Options like radical prostatectomy or high-dose radiation are considered to eliminate the cancer and reduce the risk of recurrence.

- <u>Older Patients:</u>

  - <u>Description</u>: Older patients or those with limited life expectancy may prioritize treatments that maintain quality of life and manage symptoms over those aiming for a cure.

  - <u>Treatment Choices:</u>

- <u>Less Invasive Options</u>: Treatments like active surveillance, hormone therapy, or palliative care focus on symptom management and minimizing side effects.

3. Overall Health and Comorbidities

A patient's overall health and the presence of other medical conditions (comorbidities) significantly influence treatment decisions.

- <u>Healthy Patients</u>:

  - <u>Description</u>: Those with good overall health and few comorbidities may tolerate aggressive treatments well.

  - <u>Treatment Choices</u>:

  - <u>Comprehensive Options</u>: Including surgery and intensive radiation, which may offer better outcomes in terms of cancer control.

- <u>Patients with Significant Health Issues:</u>

-     Description: Patients   with cardiovascular disease, diabetes, or other serious conditions might face higher risks from aggressive treatments.

  - Treatment Choices:

  - Conservative Approaches: Options like active surveillance or hormone therapy that pose fewer risks and complications.

4. Potential Side Effects and Quality of Life

Understanding and weighing the potential side effects of treatments is essential for making a balanced decision.

- Side Effects:

  - Urinary Incontinence: A potential side effect of surgery and radiation therapy, impacting a patient's daily activities and quality of life.

- <u>Erectile Dysfunction</u>: Common after surgery and radiation, affecting sexual health and relationships.

- <u>Bowel Problems</u>: Possible with radiation therapy, leading to discomfort and changes in bowel habits.

<u>Quality of Life Considerations:</u>

- <u>Balancing Act:</u> Patients must consider how treatment side effects will affect their overall quality of life and weigh these against the potential benefits of the treatment.

- <u>Informed Decisions:</u> Comprehensive discussions with healthcare providers about the likelihood and management of side effects can guide better decision-making.

5. Patient Preferences

Personal values and individual preferences are central to selecting a treatment plan.

- **Quality of Life vs. Aggressiveness:**

- <u>Description</u>: Some patients may prioritize treatments that offer the best chance of curing the cancer, even if they come with significant side effects. Others might prefer options that maintain a higher quality of life, even if it means less aggressive treatment.

- <u>Treatment Choices:</u>

- <u>Quality of Life Prioritization:</u> Patients may opt for active surveillance or hormone therapy to avoid the side effects of surgery and radiation.

- <u>Aggressive Treatment:</u> Patients who want to eliminate cancer entirely might choose surgery or high-dose radiation, despite the potential side effects.

- **Involvement in Decision-Making**

- <u>Empowerment</u>: Actively involving patients in discussions about their treatment options, risks, and outcomes ensures that their values and preferences are respected.

- Shared Decision-Making**: Encouraging patients to share their concerns and preferences helps create a tailored treatment plan that aligns with their goals and lifestyle.

Deciding on a treatment plan for prostate cancer involves a multifaceted assessment of the cancer's characteristics, the patient's health, potential side effects, and personal preferences. By considering these factors, patients and their healthcare providers can collaborate to choose the most suitable and effective treatment strategy. Understanding the implications of each factor helps ensure that the chosen treatment aligns with the patient's overall goals, whether aiming for a cure, maintaining quality of life, or managing symptoms. This comprehensive approach is essential for optimal prostate cancer management and patient satisfaction.

Here are the treatment options your health provider might recommend

1) Watchful Waiting or Active Surveillance

Your doctor may recommend a monitoring approach, either Watchful Waiting or Active Surveillance, to observe your tumor's progression before initiating treatment. Since most prostate cancers progress slowly, some doctors advocate for delaying treatment until the cancer shows signs of growth or causes symptoms. With Watchful Waiting, your doctor will regularly assess your symptoms and overall health. Active Surveillance takes it a step further, incorporating regular tests to closely monitor the cancer's development and adjust treatment plans accordingly."

2) **Surgery**

Surgery is a viable option if you're in good health and your cancer is localized, meaning it hasn't spread. There are various surgical approaches, including removing just the prostate gland or the gland and surrounding tissue.

Common side effects of surgery include urinary incontinence and erectile dysfunction. However, these issues may resolve on their own, especially bladder control problems. It's essential to discuss the potential risks and benefits with your surgeon beforehand, as they may be able to take steps to preserve the nerves surrounding the prostate and minimize these side effects.

3) **Radiation**

This treatment uses high-energy beams (similar to X-rays) to kill the cancer. It's often a choice when your cancer is low grade or still only in your prostate. You also might have it after surgery to get rid of any cancer cells left behind. It also helps with cancer that has spread to the bone.

There are two types of radiation therapy: external beam radiation and brachytherapy.

External: A machine outside your body directs rays at the cancer. External beam radiation therapy (EBRT) is the most common type of radiation therapy. EBRT uses CT scans and MRIs to map out the location of the tumor cells and X-rays are targeted to those areas. EBRT treatment is non-invasive and there is no down time or healing time.

Internal (brachytherapy): A doctor does surgery to place small radioactive "seeds" into or near the cancer. Brachytherapy involves placing radiation therapy "seeds" or temporary catheters inside the prostate that emit radiation at a very short distance. It is usually done in one to four treatment sessions depending on the method used.

Sometimes, a mix of both treatments works best.

4) Proton Beam Radiation

This special kind of radiation therapy uses very small particles to attack and kill cancer cells that haven't spread.

5) Radiopharmaceuticals

Radiopharmaceuticals, or medicinal radio-compounds, are a group of pharmaceutical drugs containing radioactive isotopes. This form of radiation is used to treat patients diagnosed with castration-resistant metastatic prostate cancer as a method of controlling the disease. The drugs can be taken orally or by injection. In some cases, they may be placed in the prostate itself

6) Hormone Therapy

Prostate cancer cells need male sex hormones, like testosterone, to keep growing. This treatment keeps the cancer cells from getting them. Your doctor might call it androgen deprivation therapy. Some hormone treatments lower the levels of testosterone and other male hormones. Other types block the way those hormones work.

7) Chemotherapy

Drugs that you take by mouth or through an IV travel through your body, attacking and killing cancer cells and shrinking tumors. You might get chemo if the disease has spread outside your prostate and hormone therapy isn't working for you.

8) Immunotherapy

This treatment works with your immune system to fight the disease. It's used to treat advanced prostate cancer

9) Bisphosphonate Therapy

If the disease reaches your bones, these drugs can ease pain and prevent fractures.

10) Cryotherapy or Cryosurgery

If you have early prostate cancer, your doctor might choose to kill cancer cells by freezing them. They'll put small needles or probes into your prostate to deliver very cold gasses that destroy the cells.

It's hard to say for sure how well it works. Scientists haven't done much long-term research that focuses on using it to treat prostate cancer. It's usually not the first treatment a doctor recommends

11) Prostate Cancer Vaccine:

This personalized treatment harnesses the power of your immune system to target and combat cancer cells. It's most effective when used after hormone therapy has stopped working. While its impact on cancer growth is unclear, research suggests it can help extend the lives of men living with prostate cancer. The vaccine is tailored specifically to each individual, and scientists continue to study its potential in the fight against this disease.

12) High-Intensity Focused Ultrasound

High-intensity focused ultrasound is not a standard in care but is used for patients seeking an option between active surveillance and radical therapy. This device produces sound waves that deliver heat energy to kill cancer cells. It's unclear how well it works, as it hasn't yet been compared with other standard prostate cancer treatments.

CHAPTER 6 Treatment Options for Localized Prostate Cancer

1. Active Surveillance in Prostate Cancer Management

Active surveillance is a strategic approach to managing prostate cancer that focuses on closely monitoring the disease rather than initiating immediate treatment. This method is especially suited for certain categories of patients and aims to balance effective cancer control with maintaining quality of life.

Active surveillance involves the careful and regular observation of prostate cancer through a series of medical tests and examinations. The primary objective is to keep track of the cancer's status over time and to begin treatment only if there are indications of disease progression.

The key components of active surveillance include:

1. PSA Tests: The prostate-specific antigen (PSA) test is a blood test that measures the level of PSA, a protein produced by prostate cells. Elevated levels of PSA can be an indicator of prostate cancer. During active surveillance, PSA tests are conducted regularly, typically every 3 to 6 months, to monitor any changes that might suggest the cancer is progressing.

2. Digital Rectal Exams (DREs): In this physical examination, a healthcare provider inserts a lubricated, gloved finger into the rectum to feel the prostate gland. The provider checks for any irregularities, such as lumps or hard areas, that might indicate changes in the cancer. DREs are usually performed annually as part of the active surveillance protocol.

3. **Prostate Biopsies**: Biopsies involve taking small samples of prostate tissue to examine for cancer cells under a microscope. This procedure is often guided by transrectal ultrasound (TRUS) to ensure accurate sampling. An initial biopsy is typically performed within the first year of starting active surveillance, followed by additional biopsies every 1 to 3 years depending on individual risk factors and previous biopsy results.

Who It's For

Active surveillance is particularly suitable for:

- Men with Low-Risk Prostate Cancer: This group includes patients diagnosed with cancer that has a Gleason score of 6 or lower, a PSA level below 10 ng/mL, and cancer confined to the prostate (T1-T2a stage). These factors suggest that the cancer is slow-growing and unlikely to cause significant harm in the short term.

- Men with Significant Comorbidities: For older men or those with serious health conditions such as cardiovascular disease, diabetes, or other chronic illnesses, the risks associated with aggressive treatments like surgery or radiation may outweigh the potential benefits. Active surveillance allows these patients to avoid the risks of immediate treatment while still keeping the cancer under close observation.

Benefits

The main benefits of active surveillance include:

- **Avoidance or Delay of Side Effects**: Traditional prostate cancer treatments, such as surgery (radical prostatectomy) and radiation therapy, can result in significant side effects, including urinary incontinence, erectile dysfunction, and bowel problems. By choosing active surveillance, patients can avoid or delay these adverse effects, thus maintaining a better quality of life for a longer period.

- **Quality of Life:** Many men on active surveillance can continue their normal activities without the physical and emotional toll associated with aggressive cancer treatments. This approach allows patients to live relatively unaffected by their cancer as long as it remains under control.

Risks

While active surveillance offers significant benefits, it also presents certain risks:

- **Cancer Progression**: One of the primary concerns with active surveillance is that the cancer could grow or spread during the monitoring period. If the cancer progresses undetected, it might become more difficult to treat effectively when treatment is eventually initiated.

- **Regular Follow-Up:** Active surveillance requires frequent follow-up appointments, including PSA tests, DREs, and biopsies. These regular tests can be burdensome and stressful for some patients. Additionally, the invasive nature of repeated biopsies can lead to discomfort, bleeding, and a small risk of infection.

- **Psychological Impact:** Knowing that one has cancer and choosing not to treat it immediately can cause significant anxiety and stress for some men. The uncertainty about whether the cancer might progress can affect a patient's mental health and overall well-being.

The Active Surveillance Process

The process of active surveillance is tailored to each patient's specific situation but generally follows a standard protocol:

1. Initial Monitoring Phase:

   - PSA tests every 3-6 months to monitor for any significant changes in PSA levels.

   - DREs at least once a year to physically assess the prostate.

- Biopsies within the first year of diagnosis and then every 1-3 years, depending on the results and other factors.

2. <u>Continued Monitoring</u>:

- Ongoing PSA tests and DREs at intervals determined by the patient's initial response to surveillance.

- Additional biopsies if there is a significant rise in PSA levels or if DRE findings suggest potential cancer progression.

3. Intervention:

- If tests indicate that the cancer is progressing (e.g., a significant increase in PSA, changes in DRE, or biopsy results showing higher Gleason scores or more extensive cancer), the patient and healthcare provider will discuss and initiate appropriate treatment options.

These might include surgery, radiation therapy, hormone therapy, or other modalities.

Decision-Making in Active Surveillance

Choosing active surveillance involves careful consideration and ongoing discussions between the patient and their healthcare provider. Factors to consider include:

- **Patient's Overall Health and Life Expectancy:** Younger, healthier men may opt for more aggressive treatment to eliminate the cancer, while older men with other health issues might prefer to avoid the side effects of such treatments.
- **Patient's Preferences and Anxiety Levels:** Some patients may feel comfortable with a "watchful waiting" approach, while others might find the lack

of immediate treatment stressful and prefer a more aggressive approach.

-Cancer Characteristics: Detailed information about the cancer's Gleason score, PSA levels, and staging is critical in determining if active surveillance is appropriate.

Active surveillance is a viable and increasingly popular approach for managing low-risk prostate cancer. It allows patients to avoid the side effects of aggressive treatments while maintaining close monitoring to ensure timely intervention if the cancer shows signs of progression. This strategy underscores the importance of individualized patient care, considering the patient's overall health, cancer characteristics, and personal preferences in the management plan. Through regular follow-up and advanced diagnostic tools, active surveillance provides a balanced approach to managing prostate cancer, emphasizing both quality of life and vigilant monitoring.

2. Radical Prostatectomy

Description

Radical prostatectomy is a surgical procedure aimed at treating prostate cancer by removing the entire prostate gland along with some of the surrounding tissues. This approach is often chosen for patients with localized prostate cancer where the disease has not spread beyond the prostate. The goal of the surgery is to eliminate the cancerous cells and prevent the cancer from spreading or recurring.

Types

There are several types of radical prostatectomy, each differing in technique and approach:

- **Open Radical Prostatectomy**: This is the traditional method where a surgeon makes a single, long incision in the lower abdomen to access and remove the prostate gland. This approach allows the surgeon a direct view of the prostate and surrounding tissues.

- **Laparoscopic Radical Prostatectomy**: This minimally invasive technique involves several small incisions through which the surgeon inserts a camera and surgical instruments. The camera provides a magnified view of the prostate on a screen, guiding the surgeon as they remove the prostate gland. This method generally results in less postoperative pain and a quicker recovery compared to open surgery.

- **Robotic-Assisted Laparoscopic Prostatectomy:** An advanced form of laparoscopic surgery, this method utilizes robotic technology to assist the surgeon. The surgeon controls the robotic arms, which provide enhanced precision, flexibility, and control during the procedure. The robotic system translates the surgeon's hand movements into smaller, more precise movements of the surgical instruments inside the patient's body.

Who It's For

Radical prostatectomy is typically recommended for:

- **Men with Localized Prostate Cancer:** Candidates for this surgery usually have cancer confined to the prostate gland, meaning it has not spread to other parts of the body.

- Men in Good Health: Patients should be in good overall health to tolerate the surgery and anesthesia.

- Men with a Life Expectancy of 10 Years or More: Since prostate cancer is often slow-growing, this procedure is generally recommended for patients who are expected to live at least another decade, making it likely they will benefit from the potential cure provided by the surgery.

Benefits

The primary benefits of radical prostatectomy include:

- Potentially Curative: For men with localized prostate cancer, removing the entire prostate gland can effectively eliminate the cancer. This offers a significant chance of curing the disease, especially when the cancer is detected early and has not spread.

- Comprehensive Removal: The procedure allows for the removal of the entire prostate and surrounding tissues, which helps ensure that no cancerous cells are left behind.

Risks

While radical prostatectomy can be highly effective, it also carries several risks and potential side effects:

- Urinary Incontinence: This is one of the most common side effects, where patients experience leakage of urine following the surgery. Although this often improves over time, some patients may continue to have issues with incontinence.

- Erectile Dysfunction: Nerve damage during surgery can lead to difficulties achieving or maintaining an erection. The extent of this problem can vary depending on the patient's age, baseline erectile function, and whether nerve-sparing techniques were used during surgery.

- Complications from Surgery: As with any major surgery, there are risks of complications such as infection, bleeding, blood clots, and reactions to anesthesia. Minimally invasive techniques like laparoscopic or robotic-assisted surgery tend to have fewer complications compared to open surgery.

Radical prostatectomy is a well-established treatment option for men with localized prostate cancer. By surgically removing the prostate gland and surrounding tissues, it aims to cure the disease and prevent its spread. The choice of surgical method—whether open, laparoscopic, or robotic-assisted—depends on various factors, including the patient's health, the surgeon's expertise, and the specific characteristics of the cancer. Despite its potential side effects and risks, radical prostatectomy remains a cornerstone in the treatment of prostate cancer, offering a significant chance of cure for many patients.

3. Radiation Therapy for Prostate Cancer

Description: Radiation therapy is a medical treatment that uses high-energy rays or particles to target and kill cancer cells. This treatment aims to destroy the DNA within cancer cells, preventing them from growing and dividing. Radiation therapy can be utilized as a primary treatment for prostate cancer, as well as in combination with other treatments such as surgery or hormone therapy.

Types:

1. **External Beam Radiation Therapy (EBRT)**

   - **Description**: EBRT involves directing high-energy radiation beams at the prostate gland from outside the body using a machine called a linear accelerator. Advanced techniques like Intensity-Modulated Radiation Therapy (IMRT) and Image-Guided Radiation Therapy (IGRT) allow for more precise targeting of the cancer, minimizing damage to surrounding healthy tissue.

   - **Process**: Treatment planning starts with a simulation session, where imaging tests like CT or MRI scans are used to map the exact location of the prostate and surrounding structures. Patients typically receive EBRT five days a week for several weeks, with each session lasting only a few minutes.

- **Benefits**: Non-invasive with no need for anesthesia or hospitalization. It's highly effective for treating localized prostate cancer and can be tailored to minimize exposure to nearby organs.

- **Risks**: Potential side effects include urinary issues (such as increased frequency or urgency, and discomfort during urination), bowel problems (like diarrhea, rectal bleeding, and rectal pain), and erectile dysfunction. Fatigue is also a common side effect during and after the treatment course.

2. Brachytherapy:

- Description: Brachytherapy, also known as internal radiation therapy, involves placing radioactive seeds or pellets directly into the prostate gland. These seeds emit radiation over a period of time, targeting cancer cells with high doses of radiation while limiting exposure to surrounding healthy tissue.

- Types: There are two main forms of brachytherapy for prostate cancer:

- **Low-dose-rate (LDR) brachytherapy**: Involves permanently implanting radioactive seeds in the prostate, which release radiation slowly over several months.

- **High-dose-rate (HDR) brachytherapy:** Involves temporarily placing high-intensity radioactive sources in the prostate for short periods, typically minutes to hours, before removal.

- **Process**: The procedure is usually performed under anesthesia. For LDR, the seeds are placed using needles guided by ultrasound, and for HDR, catheters are used to deliver the radioactive material temporarily. Brachytherapy can be a single treatment or combined with EBRT for more aggressive cancers.

- **Benefits**: High precision in targeting the prostate cancer, reducing the risk of damage to surrounding tissues. It's a minimally invasive option with shorter recovery times compared to surgery.

- **Risks**: Potential side effects include urinary problems (difficulty urinating or urinary retention), bowel issues (such as rectal irritation), and erectile dysfunction. There is also a small risk of the seeds migrating to other parts of the body, though this is rare.

Who It's For: Radiation therapy is suitable for men with localized or locally advanced prostate cancer. It can be a primary treatment option for early-stage cancer, an adjunct to surgery, or used in cases where cancer has recurred. It is also considered for patients who may not be ideal candidates for surgery due to other health conditions or personal preferences.

Benefits: Radiation therapy, particularly EBRT, is non-invasive and generally well-tolerated, with outpatient treatments that do not require hospital stays. It effectively targets localized cancer, potentially preserving prostate function and offering a good quality of life post-treatment. Brachytherapy provides a targeted approach with fewer sessions needed compared to EBRT, and often results in less overall radiation exposure to the body.

Risks: While radiation therapy is effective, it does come with potential side effects.

Urinary problems are common, including increased frequency, urgency, and discomfort during urination. Bowel issues, such as diarrhea, rectal bleeding, and rectal pain, may occur. Erectile dysfunction can also be a concern, with the risk varying based on the patient's age, overall health, and the specific type of radiation therapy used. Fatigue is another common side effect, which typically improves after treatment concludes.

In summary, radiation therapy offers a range of options for treating prostate cancer, from non-invasive EBRT to precise brachytherapy, each with its unique advantages and potential risks. The choice of therapy depends on various factors, including the stage of cancer, patient health, and personal preferences. Consulting with a healthcare provider specializing in cancer treatment is essential to determine the best approach for each individual case.

4.   Focal Therapy for Prostate Cancer

Focal therapy is an emerging approach in the treatment of prostate cancer that aims to target and destroy only the cancerous tissue within the prostate while sparing as much of the healthy tissue as possible. This targeted method contrasts with more traditional treatments like surgery or radiation, which affect the entire prostate and often surrounding areas. The goal of focal therapy is to reduce the side effects and complications associated with these broader treatments while effectively controlling the cancer.

Types:

1. **High-Intensity Focused Ultrasound (HIFU):**

IFU uses focused ultrasound waves to generate intense heat at a precise point within the prostate. This heat destroys the cancer cells in the targeted area. The procedure is guided by real-time imaging, usually via MRI or ultrasound, to ensure accurate targeting of the cancerous tissue.

- **Process**: The patient is typically placed under anesthesia, and a probe is inserted into the rectum to deliver the ultrasound waves. The procedure can take a few hours, depending on the size and location of the cancerous tissue. HIFU can be performed as an outpatient procedure, allowing patients to go home the same day.

- **Benefits**: Minimally invasive with no incisions required. There is a quick recovery time, often just a few days, and fewer complications compared to more invasive surgeries. HIFU is particularly beneficial in preserving urinary and sexual function.

-**Risks**: Potential side effects include urinary problems, such as difficulty urinating or incontinence, and erectile dysfunction, although these are generally less common and severe than with traditional treatments. There is also a risk of rectal fistula (an abnormal connection between the rectum and other organs), though this is rare.

2. Cryotherapy:

Cryotherapy, also known as cryoablation, involves freezing the cancer cells within the prostate. This is done by inserting thin needles or probes into the prostate and circulating extremely cold gases, such as argon or nitrogen, to freeze and destroy the targeted tissue.

- **Process**: The procedure is typically performed under anesthesia. Needles are inserted into the prostate through the perineum (the area between the scrotum and anus), guided by ultrasound or MRI imaging. The freezing process involves a cycle of freezing and thawing to ensure all targeted cells are destroyed. Patients are usually able to go home the same day or the following day.

- **Benefits**: Cryotherapy is minimally invasive and can be an effective treatment for localized prostate cancer with a relatively quick recovery period. It can also be repeated if necessary, and it is less likely to affect surrounding tissues compared to broader treatments like radiation.

- **Risks**: Side effects can include urinary incontinence, erectile dysfunction, and potential damage to the rectum or urethra. Some patients might experience swelling or discomfort in the treated area.

Appropriate Candidates: Focal therapy is generally suitable for men with low to intermediate-risk localized prostate cancer. It is often considered for patients who have cancer confined to specific areas of the prostate and who are looking for a treatment option that minimizes side effects. Ideal candidates typically have a small, well-defined tumor that has not spread beyond the prostate. Focal therapy is also an option for patients who may not be suitable candidates for more invasive treatments due to age, overall health, or personal preferences.

Benefits:

- **Minimally Invasive**:: Both HIFU and cryotherapy involve minimal incisions, leading to faster recovery times and reduced risk of infection compared to traditional surgery.

- **Fewer Side Effects**: By targeting only the cancerous tissue, focal therapy reduces the risk of common side effects associated with prostate cancer treatments, such as urinary incontinence and erectile dysfunction. This can significantly improve the patient's quality of life post-treatment.

- **Outpatient Procedure:** Many focal therapy treatments can be performed on an outpatient basis, allowing patients to return home the same day and resume normal activities more quickly.

- Potential for Repeat Treatment If cancer recurs, focal therapy can often be repeated, providing an additional treatment option without resorting to more aggressive treatments.

Risks:

- **Limited Long-Term Data**: While focal therapy shows promise, there is still limited long-term data on its effectiveness compared to traditional treatments. More research and clinical trials are needed to fully understand its long-term success rates and potential complications.

- Potential for Incomplete Cancer Eradication: Since focal therapy targets specific areas of the prostate, there is a risk that some cancer cells may be missed, leading to recurrence. Careful monitoring and follow-up are crucial to address any potential issues promptly.

- Technical Challenges: The success of focal therapy heavily relies on accurate imaging and targeting of cancerous tissue. Any inaccuracies in imaging or treatment delivery can result in incomplete treatment or damage to healthy tissue.

In conclusion, focal therapy represents a promising advancement in the treatment of prostate cancer, offering a less invasive option with fewer side effects compared to traditional treatments. While it is particularly suitable for men with localized, low to intermediate-risk prostate cancer, ongoing research and clinical trials will continue to refine these techniques and expand their applicability. As with any medical treatment, patients should discuss the potential benefits and risks with their healthcare provider to determine the best approach for their individual condition.

CHAPTER 7: Treatment Options for Advanced Prostate Cancer

I) Hormonal Therapy (Androgen Deprivation Therapy - ADT) for Prostate Cancer

Hormonal therapy, also known as Androgen Deprivation Therapy (ADT), is a treatment designed to reduce levels of male hormones, or androgens, in the body. Androgens, particularly testosterone, can stimulate the growth of prostate cancer cells. By lowering androgen levels or blocking their effects, ADT can help slow the progression of prostate cancer and alleviate symptoms.

Types

1. LHRH Agonists:

LHRH (Luteinizing Hormone-Releasing Hormone) agonists, also known as GnRH (Gonadotropin-Releasing Hormone) agonists, work by initially increasing the production of luteinizing hormone, which temporarily raises testosterone levels before drastically reducing them. This process, known as a "flare," is followed by a significant drop in testosterone production as the testes stop producing the hormone.

- **Examples**: Leuprolide (Lupron), Goserelin (Zoladex), Triptorelin (Trelstar).

-**Administration**: These drugs are typically administered via injection, either monthly, quarterly, or yearly, depending on the specific medication and treatment plan.

- **Benefits**: Effective in significantly reducing testosterone levels, which can help control the growth and spread of prostate cancer.

-**Risks**: Initial flare of testosterone can temporarily worsen symptoms. Common side effects include hot flashes, reduced libido, fatigue, and bone thinning. Long-term use may also increase the risk of cardiovascular problems and diabetes.

2. LHRH Antagonists:

LHRH antagonists, or GnRH antagonists, work by directly blocking the signals from the pituitary gland that stimulate testosterone production. Unlike LHRH agonists, they do not cause an initial flare of testosterone levels.

-**Examples**: Degarelix (Firmagon), Relugolix (Orgovyx).

-Administration: Degarelix is administered as a monthly injection, while Relugolix is taken as a daily oral pill.

-Benefits: Quickly reduces testosterone levels without the initial flare, making it particularly useful for patients with advanced prostate cancer and those with severe symptoms.

-Risks: Similar to LHRH agonists, side effects include hot flashes, reduced libido, fatigue, and bone thinning. There may also be injection site reactions with Degarelix.

3.Anti-Androgens:

Anti-androgens work by blocking the action of testosterone at the receptor level within prostate cancer cells. They are often used in combination with LHRH agonists or antagonists to provide a more comprehensive androgen blockade.

-**Examples**: Bicalutamide (Casodex), Flutamide (Eulexin), Enzalutamide (Xtandi), Apalutamide (Erleada).

-**Administration**: These medications are taken orally, usually once daily.

-**Benefits**: Can enhance the effectiveness of LHRH agonists or antagonists, reducing testosterone-driven cancer growth. Anti-androgens can also be used as monotherapy in certain cases.

-Risks: Side effects may include breast tenderness or enlargement, hot flashes, gastrointestinal issues, and liver toxicity. Enzalutamide and Apalutamide may also cause seizures, though this is rare.

Suitable Candidates: Hormonal therapy is primarily used for men with advanced or metastatic prostate cancer. It is also considered for patients whose cancer has returned after initial treatment or for those with high-risk localized cancer as part of a combination therapy. Additionally, ADT can be used to shrink tumors before radiation therapy or to control symptoms in men who cannot undergo surgery or other treatments.

Benefits:

-Slows Cancer Growth: By reducing androgen levels, ADT can slow the progression of prostate cancer, potentially extending survival and improving quality of life.

-Symptom Reduction: Can help alleviate symptoms associated with advanced prostate cancer, such as bone pain and urinary obstruction, enhancing patient comfort.

-Combination Therapy: Often used in conjunction with other treatments, such as radiation therapy or chemotherapy, to improve outcomes.

Risks:

- Hormonal Side Effects: Common side effects include hot flashes, reduced libido, erectile dysfunction, and fatigue. These symptoms result from the body's reduced androgen levels and can impact the patient's quality of life.

-Bone Thinning: ADT can lead to decreased bone density, increasing the risk of fractures and osteoporosis. Patients may require additional treatments to protect bone health.

-Metabolic Changes: Long-term use of ADT can lead to weight gain, insulin resistance, and an increased risk of cardiovascular diseases and diabetes.

-Emotional and Cognitive Effects: Some patients may experience mood swings, depression, and cognitive changes due to hormonal alterations.

In summary, hormonal therapy is a cornerstone treatment for advanced and metastatic prostate cancer, offering significant benefits in controlling disease progression and alleviating symptoms. However, it comes with notable side effects that require careful management and monitoring. Patients should work closely with their healthcare providers to weigh the benefits and risks and to develop a personalized treatment plan that best meets their needs.

II) Chemotherapy for Prostate Cancer

Chemotherapy is a systemic cancer treatment that uses drugs to kill rapidly dividing cancer cells throughout the body. Unlike localized treatments like surgery or radiation, which target specific areas, chemotherapy circulates through the bloodstream, attacking cancer cells wherever they may be. The drugs used in chemotherapy are designed to interfere with the cancer cells' ability to grow and divide, ultimately leading to their destruction.

Appropriate Candidates: Chemotherapy is typically used for men with advanced prostate cancer that is resistant to hormone therapy (also known as castration-resistant prostate cancer). It is also considered for patients with metastatic prostate cancer that has spread to other parts of the body, such as the bones or lymph nodes. Additionally, chemotherapy may be recommended for patients who have not responded to other treatments or as part of a combination therapy approach.

Benefits::

- Tumor Shrinkage: Chemotherapy can effectively shrink tumors, which can help relieve pain and other symptoms caused by the cancer pressing on nearby organs and tissues.

- Symptom Relief: By reducing the size of tumors, chemotherapy can alleviate symptoms such as bone pain, difficulty urinating, and other complications associated with advanced prostate cancer.

-Improved Survival: For some patients, chemotherapy can extend survival and improve the quality of life by slowing the progression of the disease.

- Combination Therapy: Chemotherapy is often used in combination with other treatments, such as hormone therapy or targeted therapy, to enhance overall effectiveness and provide a more comprehensive approach to managing the cancer.

Risks:

- **Nausea and Vomiting:** Chemotherapy drugs can irritate the stomach lining, leading to nausea and vomiting. Anti-nausea medications are often prescribed to help manage these side effects.

-**Hair Loss:** Chemotherapy can cause hair loss, as it affects rapidly dividing cells, including those responsible for hair growth. Hair typically grows back after treatment ends.

- **Fatigue**: Many patients experience significant fatigue during chemotherapy, which can impact daily activities and overall quality of life. Rest and supportive care can help manage this side effect.

- **Increased Risk of Infection::** Chemotherapy can lower white blood cell counts, weakening the immune system and increasing the risk of infections. Patients are closely monitored, and preventive measures are taken to reduce infection risks.

- **Other Side Effect**: Additional side effects can include anemia (low red blood cell counts), thrombocytopenia (low platelet counts), mouth sores, loss of appetite, and changes in taste. Long-term effects might include nerve damage (neuropathy), which can cause numbness or tingling in the hands and feet.

Common Chemotherapy Drugs for Prostate Cancer:

- **Docetaxel (Taxotere**) Often the first-line chemotherapy drug for advanced prostate cancer, typically administered every three weeks. It is sometimes combined with prednisone, a steroid that can help reduce inflammation and manage side effects.

-**Cabazitaxel (Jevtana):** Used for patients whose cancer has progressed after treatment with docetaxel. It is administered similarly to docetaxel and can provide additional options for those with resistant disease.

Administration: Chemotherapy is usually given in cycles, with a period of treatment followed by a period of rest to allow the body to recover. The specific schedule and duration of chemotherapy depend on the type of drugs used, the stage of the cancer, and the patient's overall health. Chemotherapy can be administered intravenously (through an IV) in a clinic or hospital setting, and patients are monitored for any adverse reactions during and after the infusion.

Monitoring and Support Throughout chemotherapy treatment, patients undergo regular blood tests and imaging studies to monitor the cancer's response to therapy and manage side effects. Supportive care measures, such as medications to boost blood cell counts, anti-nausea drugs, and pain management strategies, are crucial to maintaining the patient's quality of life during treatment.

Chemotherapy plays a critical role in the management of advanced and hormone-resistant prostate cancer. While it comes with a range of potential side effects, the benefits of tumor shrinkage, symptom relief, and potential improvement in survival can make it a valuable treatment option. Patients should have thorough discussions with their oncologists to understand the potential benefits and risks, explore supportive care options, and develop a personalized treatment plan that aligns with their health status and treatment goals.

III. Targeted Therapy for Prostate Cancer

Targeted therapy is a form of cancer treatment that uses drugs designed to specifically target cancer cells with certain genetic mutations or abnormalities. Unlike traditional chemotherapy, which affects all rapidly dividing cells, targeted therapy aims to interfere with specific molecules involved in the growth, progression, and spread of cancer cells. This precision approach allows for more effective treatment with potentially fewer side effects, as it spares normal, healthy cells.

Types:

1. PARP Inhibitors:

   - Description: PARP (Poly ADP-ribose Polymerase) inhibitors are a class of targeted therapy drugs that interfere with the PARP enzyme, which helps repair DNA damage in cells. Cancer cells with BRCA1 or BRCA2 mutations rely heavily on PARP for DNA repair. By inhibiting this enzyme, PARP inhibitors cause the accumulation of DNA damage in these cancer cells, leading to their death.

-**Eamples**: Olaparib (Lynparza) and Rucaparib (Rubraca).

- **Mechanism of Action:** PARP inhibitors block the PARP enzyme's activity, preventing cancer cells from repairing their damaged DNA. This action is particularly effective in cells that already have defects in other DNA repair mechanisms, such as those with BRCA mutations. The inability to repair DNA damage ultimately leads to the death of these cancer cells.

-*

Administration: PARP inhibitors are typically administered orally in pill form. The dosage and treatment schedule depend on the specific drug and the patient's overall treatment plan.

Suitable Candidates: Targeted therapy, specifically PARP inhibitors, is suitable for men with advanced prostate cancer who have specific genetic profiles. This includes patients with mutations in the BRCA1 or BRCA2 genes, as well as other mutations affecting DNA repair pathways. Genetic testing is essential to identify patients who would benefit most from targeted therapy. It is particularly used for those whose cancer has progressed despite other treatments, such as hormone therapy or chemotherapy.

Benefits:

- **Precision Treatment**: Targeted therapy directly attacks cancer cells with specific genetic mutations, sparing normal cells and potentially reducing side effects compared to traditional chemotherapy.
- Effective for Resistant Cancers Targeted therapy can be particularly effective for cancers that have become resistant to other treatments, providing an important option for patients with advanced disease.
- **Oral Administration**:: Many targeted therapy drugs, including PARP inhibitors, are taken orally, making them more convenient and less invasive than treatments requiring intravenous administration.

Risks:

- **Side Effects**: While targeted therapies are generally better tolerated than traditional chemotherapy, they are not without side effects. Common side effects of PARP inhibitors include fatigue, nausea, vomiting, diarrhea, and loss of appetite. Some patients may experience more severe side effects, such as blood disorders (e.g., anemia, low white blood cell counts), liver enzyme abnormalities, and potential increased risk of infections.

- Development of Resistance: Cancer cells can develop resistance to targeted therapies over time, necessitating changes in treatment strategy. Ongoing monitoring and adjustments are crucial to manage resistance.

- **Genetic** Testing Requirement: The effectiveness of targeted therapy depends on identifying the right genetic mutations. This requires comprehensive genetic testing, which may not be accessible to all patients and can delay the start of treatment.

Monitoring and Management: Patients undergoing targeted therapy need regular monitoring to assess the effectiveness of the treatment and manage any side effects. This typically involves periodic blood tests, imaging studies, and clinical evaluations. Healthcare providers may adjust the dosage or switch medications based on the patient's response and any side effects encountered.

Targeted therapy represents a significant advancement in the treatment of prostate cancer, particularly for those with specific genetic mutations such as BRCA1 or BRCA2. By focusing on the unique characteristics of cancer cells, targeted therapy offers the potential for more effective treatment with fewer side effects. However, it requires thorough genetic testing to identify suitable candidates and careful management to address any emerging resistance or side effects. Patients should work closely with their healthcare team to understand the potential benefits and risks and to develop a personalized treatment plan that aligns with their genetic profile and treatment history.

IV) Immunotherapy for Prostate Cancer

Immunotherapy is a cutting-edge cancer treatment that harnesses and enhances the body's own immune system to fight cancer. Unlike traditional treatments that directly target and kill cancer cells, immunotherapy works by stimulating the immune system to recognize and destroy cancer cells more effectively. This approach can lead to durable and long-lasting responses by equipping the immune system to combat cancer more efficiently.

Types

1. Sipuleucel-T (Provenge):

Sipuleucel-T, marketed under the brand name Provenge, is an autologous cellular immunotherapy specifically designed for prostate cancer. It is a therapeutic vaccine, meaning it is used to treat existing cancer rather than prevent it. Provenge stimulates the patient's immune system to target and attack prostate cancer cells.

- **Mechanism of Action:** Provenge involves collecting a patient's own immune cells, modifying them to enhance their ability to target prostate cancer cells, and then reinfusing them back into the patient.

This process begins with leukapheresis, where immune cells are harvested from the patient's blood. These cells are then exposed to a protein that is found on most prostate cancer cells (prostatic acid phosphatase) and a substance that boosts immune responses. The activated immune cells are then returned to the patient's bloodstream, where they help stimulate the body's immune response against prostate cancer cells.

- **Administration**: The treatment involves three infusions given approximately two weeks apart. Each infusion follows a leukapheresis procedure to collect the immune cells.

Appropriate Candidates: Sipuleucel-T is typically recommended for men with advanced prostate cancer that is no longer responding to hormone therapy, also known as castration-resistant prostate cancer (CRPC). It is generally used for patients who have minimal or no symptoms and whose cancer has spread but remains confined to the prostate and surrounding areas. Genetic testing and careful patient selection are crucial to identify those who are most likely to benefit from this treatment.

Benefits:

- Prolonged Survival: Clinical trials have shown that Sipuleucel-T can extend the survival of men with advanced prostate cancer. While it may not significantly reduce tumor size or PSA levels, it can enhance the body's immune response, leading to longer-term benefits.

-Fewer Side Effects: Compared to traditional chemotherapy, Provenge is associated with fewer and generally less severe side effects. This makes it a more tolerable option for many patients, improving their quality of life during treatment.

-Personalized Treatment:: As an autologous therapy, Provenge is tailored to each individual patient, using their own immune cells to fight cancer.

Risks:

- cute Infusion Reactions Some patients may experience side effects related to the infusion process. Common side effects include fever, chills, and fatigue, which usually occur shortly after the infusion and resolve within a few days.

- **Systemic Symptoms**: Other potential side effects include headache, nausea, and joint pain. These symptoms are typically mild to moderate in severity.

- **Rare Serious Reactions**: While uncommon, there can be more serious side effects such as strokes. Patients are monitored closely for any adverse reactions during and after each infusion.

Monitoring and Management: Patients receiving Sipuleucel-T require regular follow-up to monitor their response to the treatment and manage any side effects. This involves periodic blood tests, imaging studies, and clinical evaluations to ensure the therapy is working as intended and to address any complications that arise. Supportive care measures, such as medications to manage fever and pain, are often used to help alleviate side effects and improve patient comfort.

Immunotherapy, particularly with Sipuleucel-T (Provenge), represents a significant advancement in the treatment of advanced prostate cancer. By leveraging the body's own immune system,

Provenge offers a unique and personalized approach to fighting cancer, with the potential to prolong survival and improve quality of life. While it is not without risks, the side effects are generally fewer and less severe compared to traditional chemotherapy. Patients should have thorough discussions with their healthcare providers to understand the potential benefits and risks of immunotherapy, explore whether they are suitable candidates, and develop a comprehensive treatment plan tailored to their specific needs and circumstances.

V) Radiopharmaceuticals for Prostate Cancer

Radiopharmaceuticals are a class of treatment that uses radioactive substances to target and kill cancer cells, particularly those that have spread to the bones. These drugs are designed to deliver radiation directly to the cancer cells while minimizing exposure to the surrounding healthy tissues. By mimicking natural substances that the body uses to build bone, radiopharmaceuticals can effectively target areas of bone metastasis, providing both therapeutic and palliative benefits.

Types

1. Radium-223 (Xofigo):

Radium-223 dichloride, marketed under the brand name Xofigo, is a radiopharmaceutical specifically approved for the treatment of metastatic prostate cancer with symptomatic bone metastases. Radium-223 is an alpha-emitting radiopharmaceutical, which means it releases alpha particles, a type of radiation that has a high energy but a very short range. This property allows Radium-223 to deliver powerful radiation directly to the site of bone metastases with minimal impact on surrounding healthy tissue.

- **Mechanism of Action**: Radium-223 mimics calcium, a mineral that naturally targets bone tissue. When administered, Radium-223 is absorbed by bone, particularly in areas where bone is being remodeled due to cancer metastases. The alpha particles emitted by Radium-223 cause double-strand breaks in the DNA of nearby cancer cells, leading to their death. This targeted approach helps to reduce the tumor burden in the bones and alleviate associated symptoms.

- **Administration**: Radium-223 is administered via intravenous injection, typically once every four weeks for up to six cycles. The dosage and schedule are determined based on the patient's overall health, extent of bone metastases, and response to treatment.

Appropriate Candidates: Radiopharmaceuticals like Radium-223 are primarily indicated for men with advanced prostate cancer that has spread to the bones but not to other organs. These patients often experience significant bone pain and other complications due to bone metastases. Radium-223 is particularly suitable for men with castration-resistant prostate cancer (CRPC), where the cancer has progressed despite hormone therapy.

Benefits:

- **Bone Pain Relief**: One of the most significant benefits of Radium-223 is its ability to relieve bone pain associated with metastases. By targeting and destroying cancer cells in the bones, it helps to reduce inflammation and pressure on the bones, improving the patient's quality of life.

- Extended Survival: Clinical studies have shown that Radium-223 can extend overall survival in men with metastatic prostate cancer. By effectively targeting bone metastases, it slows the progression of the disease and helps patients live longer.

- Improved Quality of Life: In addition to pain relief and extended survival, Radium-223 can improve other aspects of life for patients with bone metastases, including better mobility and reduced need for pain medications.

Risks:

- Nausea: Some patients may experience nausea as a side effect of Radium-223 treatment. This can often be managed with anti-nausea medications prescribed by the healthcare provider.

- **Diarrhea:** Another potential side effect is diarrhea, which may require dietary adjustments and medication to manage effectively.

- **Low Blood Cell Counts**: Radium-223 can cause a decrease in blood cell counts, including red blood cells, white blood cells, and platelets. This can lead to anemia, increased risk of infections, and bleeding problems. Regular blood tests are necessary to monitor blood cell levels and ensure patient safety.

- **Other Side Effects** Patients may also experience fatigue, swelling of the legs, or mild kidney problems. It is essential for patients to report any unusual symptoms to their healthcare provider promptly.

Monitoring and Management: Patients receiving Radium-223 require careful monitoring to assess the treatment's effectiveness and manage side effects. This typically includes regular blood tests to check blood cell counts, kidney function, and other vital parameters. Imaging studies may also be performed to evaluate the response of bone metastases to the treatment. Supportive care measures, such as medications to manage side effects and nutritional support, are often necessary to help patients cope with the treatment and maintain their quality of life.

Radiopharmaceuticals like Radium-223 (Xofigo) represent a powerful option for men with advanced prostate cancer that has spread to the bones. By delivering targeted radiation to bone metastases, these treatments can effectively relieve pain, improve quality of life, and extend survival. While they come with potential risks and side effects, careful monitoring and supportive care can help manage these issues. Patients considering radiopharmaceuticals should have thorough discussions with their healthcare team to understand the potential benefits and risks, ensuring that they receive personalized and comprehensive care tailored to their specific needs and circumstances.

Emerging And Experimental Treatments

1. Gene Therapy for Prostate Cancer

Gene therapy is an innovative and experimental approach to treating cancer that involves altering the genetic material within a patient's cells to fight or prevent disease. In the context of prostate cancer, gene therapy aims to modify the genes inside cancer cells to stop their growth, induce cancer cell death, or make the cancer cells more susceptible to other treatments. This can be achieved by introducing new genes into the cancer cells, repairing mutated genes, or altering the expression of existing genes.

Mechanisms of Action:

1. Gene Addition: Introducing new genes into cancer cells to produce proteins that inhibit cancer cell growth or induce cell death. For example, inserting genes that produce tumor-suppressing proteins can help control or eliminate cancer.

2. Gene Editing: Using technologies like CRISPR/Cas9 to directly edit the DNA of cancer cells. This can involve correcting mutations that cause cancer or disrupting genes essential for cancer cell survival.

3. Gene Silencing: Using RNA interference (RNAi) or other methods to silence specific genes that promote cancer cell growth and survival. By turning off these oncogenes, the growth of cancer can be slowed or stopped.

4. Immune System Enhancement: Modifying immune cells with genetic changes to better recognize and attack prostate cancer cells. This approach can make the body's immune response more effective against cancer.

Current Research: Ongoing clinical trials and research are investigating a variety of gene therapy approaches for prostate cancer. Some notable areas of research include:

1.Oncolytic Viruses:
These are genetically modified viruses designed to selectively infect and kill cancer cells while sparing normal cells. Oncolytic viruses can also stimulate an immune response against cancer.

Curren Status: Clinical trials are evaluating the safety and efficacy of oncolytic viruses in treating prostate cancer. Early results are promising, showing the potential to reduce tumor size and improve patient outcomes.

2.)CAR-T Cell Therapy

-This involves extracting a patient's T cells (a type of immune cell), genetically modifying them to express Chimeric Antigen Receptors (CARs) that recognize prostate cancer cells, and then infusing the modified T cells back into the patient. These CAR-T cells can then target and destroy cancer cells more effectively.

- **Current Status:** CAR-T cell therapy has shown remarkable success in treating certain blood cancers and is now being adapted for solid tumors like prostate cancer. Clinical trials are ongoing to determine the best ways to use CAR-T cells for prostate cancer treatment.

3. Gene Transfer:

- This approach involves transferring genes into prostate cancer cells using vectors such as viruses. The new genes can either promote cell death or inhibit cell division and tumor growth.

- **Current Status**: Various gene transfer techniques are being tested in clinical trials, with researchers exploring different vectors and gene targets to optimize treatment outcomes.

4. Gene Editing Technologies:

-Techniques like CRISPR/Cas9 allow precise editing of the DNA in prostate cancer cells. This can involve correcting cancer-causing mutations or disabling genes that drive cancer growth.

- **Current Status**: Research is still in early stages, with preclinical studies showing the potential of gene editing to treat prostate cancer. Clinical trials will be necessary to ensure safety and efficacy in humans.

Challenges and Considerations:

While gene therapy holds great promise, there are several challenges and considerations:

-**Delivery Methods** Effective and safe delivery of genetic material to the target cells remains a major hurdle. Researchers are exploring various vectors, including viral and non-viral systems, to improve delivery efficiency and reduce potential side effects.

- **Immune Response**: The body's immune system may recognize and attack the introduced genetic material or the vectors used to deliver it, which can limit the effectiveness of gene therapy. Strategies to modulate the immune response are under investigation.

- **Off-Target Effects**: Ensuring that gene therapy precisely targets cancer cells without affecting normal cells is crucial. Off-target effects can lead to unintended genetic changes, which may cause additional health issues.

- **Long-Term Effects**: The long-term effects of gene therapy are not yet fully understood. Ongoing monitoring and follow-up studies are necessary to assess the durability and safety

Gene therapy represents a revolutionary approach to treating prostate cancer, offering the potential to directly target and modify the genetic underpinnings of the disease. While still largely experimental, ongoing research and clinical trials are making significant strides in developing effective gene therapy strategies. These advancements could provide new, powerful options for patients with prostate cancer, particularly those with advanced or treatment-resistant forms of the disease. As research progresses, gene therapy may become an integral part of the oncology landscape, providing hope for more effective and personalized cancer treatments. Patients interested in gene therapy should discuss the latest research and clinical trial opportunities with their healthcare providers to explore whether these cutting-edge treatments may be suitable for their condition.

CHAPTER 8: Personalized Medicine for Prostate Cancer

Personalized medicine, also known as precision medicine, is an innovative approach to cancer treatment that involves tailoring medical care to the individual characteristics of each patient's cancer. This strategy leverages genetic testing and molecular profiling to understand the specific genetic makeup and unique molecular features of a patient's cancer. By doing so, personalized medicine aims to select the most effective treatments for each patient, thereby improving outcomes and minimizing unnecessary side effects.

Mechanisms and Strategies:

1. Genetic Testing: This involves analyzing a patient's DNA to identify mutations and alterations that drive cancer growth. These genetic insights can reveal which targeted therapies or treatments are most likely to be effective.

2. Molecular Profiling: Molecular profiling assesses the expression of genes, proteins, and other molecules in the tumor. This comprehensive analysis helps identify biomarkers that can predict a patient's response to specific treatments.

3. Biomarker Identification: Biomarkers are biological indicators, such as specific gene mutations or protein levels, that can guide treatment decisions. For example, the presence of BRCA1/2 mutations might indicate a potential benefit from PARP inhibitors.

4. Targeted Therapies: Personalized medicine often involves the use of targeted therapies, which are drugs designed to specifically inhibit cancer cells with certain genetic mutations or abnormal protein expressions.

Current Research:

Advances in genetic testing and molecular profiling are significantly advancing the field of personalized medicine for prostate cancer. Some key areas of research include:

1. Next-Generation Sequencing (NGS):

NGS technology allows for comprehensive analysis of a patient's cancer genome. This high-throughput sequencing can identify a wide range of genetic alterations, including point mutations, insertions, deletions, and copy number variations.

- **Current Status**: NGS is increasingly used in clinical settings to guide treatment decisions. Ongoing research aims to refine NGS techniques and make them more accessible and affordable for routine clinical use.

2. Liquid Biopsies

Liquid biopsies are non-invasive tests that analyze circulating tumor DNA (ctDNA) or other cancer-related molecules in the blood. These tests can provide real-time insights into the genetic makeup of a patient's cancer without the need for invasive tissue biopsies.

- **Current Status** Liquid biopsies are being investigated in clinical trials for their ability to monitor treatment response, detect resistance mutations, and guide therapy adjustments. Early results show promise for their use in personalized treatment plans.

3. Pharmacogenomics

This field studies how a patient's genetic makeup affects their response to drugs. By understanding these genetic factors, healthcare providers can choose medications that are more likely to be effective and have fewer side effects.

- **Current Status**: Pharmacogenomic testing is being integrated into clinical practice, with ongoing research focused on expanding the range of actionable genetic markers.

4. Combination Therapies:

Personalized medicine often involves combining multiple treatments tailored to the genetic and molecular profile of the cancer. This can include combinations of targeted therapies, immunotherapies, and traditional treatments like chemotherapy or radiation.

- **Current Status**: Clinical trials are exploring various combination regimens to identify the most effective treatment strategies for different genetic profiles.

Benefits

- **Improved Treatment Efficacy:** Personalized medicine increases the likelihood of treatment success by matching therapies to the specific genetic and molecular characteristics of a patient's cancer.

- **Reduced Side Effects**: By targeting only the cancer cells with specific abnormalities, personalized treatments can minimize damage to healthy cells, leading to fewer and less severe side effects.

-   **Enhanced Prognosis**: Tailored treatments can lead to better overall outcomes, including prolonged survival and improved quality of life.

- **Early Detection of Resistance**: Ongoing monitoring through techniques like liquid biopsies can detect resistance mutations early, allowing for timely adjustments to the treatment plan.

Challenges and Consideration:

- Accessibility and Cost payment for the Genetic testing and advanced molecular profiling can be expensive and may not be readily available to all patients. Efforts are underway to make these technologies more affordable and accessible.

- Complexity of Data Interpretation: The vast amount of genetic data generated by modern sequencing technologies requires sophisticated bioinformatics tools and expertise to interpret. Healthcare providers must stay updated with the latest advancements to effectively use this information.

- **Ethical and Privacy Concerns:** The collection and use of genetic information raise ethical and privacy concerns. Safeguards must be in place to protect patient data and ensure informed consent.

- **Treatment Availability:** Not all personalized treatment options are available for every type of genetic alteration identified. Continued research and development are needed to expand the arsenal of targeted therapies.

Conclusion Personalized medicine represents a transformative approach to prostate cancer treatment, offering the potential for more precise, effective, and individualized care. By harnessing the power of genetic testing and molecular profiling, personalized medicine aims to optimize treatment outcomes, minimize side effects, and improve the overall prognosis for patients. As research continues to advance, personalized medicine is expected to become increasingly integral to cancer care, providing hope for better and more tailored treatment strategies. Patients interested in personalized medicine should discuss the latest options and developments with their healthcare providers to determine the most appropriate course of action based on their specific genetic and molecular profile.

CHAPTER 9: Combination Therapy for Prostate Cancer

Combination therapy involves the use of multiple treatment modalities simultaneously or sequentially to enhance the overall effectiveness of cancer treatment. This approach aims to leverage the strengths of different treatments, targeting cancer cells through various mechanisms and reducing the likelihood of resistance. By combining therapies, healthcare providers can potentially achieve better control of cancer growth, improve patient outcomes, and prolong survival.

Mechanisms and Strategies:

1. **Surgery**: The physical removal of the prostate gland (prostatectomy) or other affected tissues. Surgery is often the first line of treatment for localized prostate cancer.

2. **Radiation Therapy:** Uses high-energy rays or particles to destroy cancer cells. Radiation can be delivered externally (External Beam Radiation Therapy, EBRT) or internally (brachytherapy).

3. **Hormone Therapy (Androgen Deprivation Therapy - ADT):** Reduces levels of male hormones (androgens) that stimulate prostate cancer growth. It can be used before, during, or after other treatments to enhance effectiveness.

4. **Chemotherapy:** Uses drugs to kill rapidly dividing cancer cells. It is often used for advanced prostate cancer that is resistant to hormone therapy.

5. Immunotherapy: Stimulates the body's immune system to recognize and attack cancer cells. This can include vaccines and immune checkpoint inhibitors.

Current Research:

Ongoing studies are exploring various combinations of these treatments to determine the most effective strategies for different stages and types of prostate cancer. Key areas of research include:

1. Surgery and Radiation Therapy:

Combining surgery with radiation therapy can help ensure that any remaining cancer cells are destroyed. This approach is particularly useful in cases where the cancer has spread beyond the prostate gland.

- **Current Status:** Clinical trials are evaluating the timing and sequencing of surgery and radiation to optimize outcomes. For instance, adjuvant radiation therapy (radiation after surgery) is being studied to see if it reduces the risk of recurrence more effectively than surgery alone.

2. Hormone Therapy and Radiation Therapy:

Hormone therapy can be used in conjunction with radiation therapy to shrink the prostate and make cancer cells more susceptible to radiation. This combination is often used for high-risk localized or locally advanced prostate cancer.

- **Current Status**: Research is focused on the optimal duration and timing of hormone therapy in relation to radiation therapy. Studies are also investigating whether combining these treatments can improve long-term survival and reduce the risk of metastasis.

3. Chemotherapy and Hormone Therapy: Chemotherapy can be combined with hormone therapy to treat advanced or metastatic prostate cancer. This combination can help overcome resistance to hormone therapy and target cancer cells more aggressively.

- **Current Status**: Ongoing trials are assessing the benefits of adding chemotherapy early in the treatment course for patients with high-risk or hormone-resistant prostate cancer. The goal is to determine whether this approach can extend survival and improve quality of life.

4. Immunotherapy and Other Treatments:

Combining immunotherapy with other treatments like radiation or hormone therapy can potentially enhance the immune response against cancer cells. For example, radiation can increase the visibility of cancer cells to the immune system, making immunotherapy more effective.

- **Current Status**: Clinical trials are exploring various combinations of immunotherapy with other modalities to identify synergies and improve outcomes. Researchers are particularly interested in understanding how these combinations can help patients who do not respond to standard treatments.

Benefits:

- Enhanced Effectiveness: Combining different treatments can attack cancer cells from multiple angles, increasing the chances of eliminating the cancer or controlling its growth.

- **Reduced Resistance**: Using multiple therapies can help prevent or delay the development of resistance, a common challenge in cancer treatment.

- **Tailored Treatment Plans**: Combination therapy allows for more personalized treatment plans, taking into account the specific characteristics of a patient's cancer and overall health.

- **Improved Survival Rates**: Studies have shown that combination therapies can improve overall survival rates for patients with prostate cancer, particularly those with advanced disease.

Challenges and Considerations:

- **Side Effects**: Combining multiple treatments can increase the risk and severity of side effects. Managing these side effects requires careful planning and supportive care.

- **Complexity of Treatment**: Coordinating and sequencing multiple treatments can be complex and requires close collaboration among healthcare providers from different specialties.

- **Individual Variation**: The effectiveness of combination therapies can vary widely among patients. Genetic and molecular profiling can help identify which combinations are most likely to be effective for individual patients.

- **Cost and Accessibility:** Combination therapies can be expensive and may not be covered by all insurance plans. Access to advanced treatments and clinical trials may also be limited.

Combination therapy represents a comprehensive and promising approach to the treatment of prostate cancer. By integrating multiple modalities, healthcare providers can create more effective and personalized treatment plans that address the unique challenges of each patient's cancer. Ongoing research continues to refine these strategies, seeking to maximize benefits while minimizing risks and side effects. Patients considering combination therapy should have detailed discussions with their healthcare team to understand the potential benefits and risks, ensuring that they receive the most appropriate and effective care tailored to their specific needs and circumstances.

.

Making Treatment Decisions

1. Consulting with Specialists:

   - It is crucial to consult with a team of healthcare providers, including urologists, oncologists, radiologists, and pathologists, to get a comprehensive view of the available options.

2. Considering Clinical Trials:

- Patients may have the opportunity to participate in clinical trials that offer access to new treatments not yet widely available.

3. Evaluating Risks and Benefits:

- Each treatment option comes with its risks and benefits. Understanding these and discussing them with healthcare providers can help patients make informed decisions.

4. Seeking Support and Second Opinions:

- It can be helpful to seek support from patient advocacy groups, support networks, and even second opinions to gain different perspectives on treatment options.

Navigating the array of treatment options for prostate cancer can be daunting. Each patient's journey is unique, and the choice of treatment should be based on a thorough understanding of the available options, the stage and grade of the cancer, and the patient's overall health and preferences. This chapter has provided a detailed overview of the various treatments, from active surveillance to advanced therapies, to help patients and their families make informed decisions about managing prostate cancer. As research and technology continue to advance, new and improved treatments will emerge, offering hope and better outcomes for those diagnosed with this disease.

CHAPTER 10: How to Move Forward: Survivorship

Survivorship encompasses the physical, emotional, and psychological aspects of life after cancer treatment. It's a critical phase where patients transition from active treatment to living beyond cancer, often facing new challenges and learning to navigate their post-cancer journey. This chapter delves into the various components of prostate cancer survivorship, offering guidance on managing health, coping with emotional changes, and finding support and purpose in the post-treatment phase.

Understanding Survivorship

Survivorship begins the moment a person is diagnosed with cancer and continues through the remainder of life. It includes the experience of living with, through, and beyond cancer. For prostate cancer survivors, the journey can be complex and multifaceted, involving ongoing health monitoring, managing long-term side effects, and adjusting to changes in lifestyle and identity.

Physical Health Management

1. Follow-Up Care and Monitoring:

- **Regular Check-Ups**: Regular medical appointments are crucial to monitor for any signs of cancer recurrence and to manage any lingering side effects of treatment. This typically includes PSA tests, digital rectal exams, and imaging tests as needed.

   - **Surveillance Protocols**: Adhering to a structured surveillance protocol helps in early detection of any potential recurrence, ensuring timely intervention.

2. Managing Long-Term Side Effects:

   - **Urinary Issues**: Incontinence or urinary difficulties can persist after treatment. Pelvic floor exercises, medications, and, in some cases, additional procedures may be needed to manage these issues.

   - **Sexual Health**: Erectile dysfunction is a common side effect. Options for management include medications (like Viagra), penile injections, vacuum erection devices, and counseling for psychological support.

- **Bowel Function**: Treatments like radiation can affect bowel function, causing issues like diarrhea or rectal bleeding. Dietary adjustments, medications, and regular follow-ups with a gastroenterologist can help manage these symptoms.

3. Healthy Lifestyle Choices:

- **Nutrition**: A balanced diet rich in fruits, vegetables, lean proteins, and whole grains supports overall health and recovery. Limiting red meat and processed foods can also reduce the risk of recurrence.

- **Exercise**: Regular physical activity helps improve physical function, reduce fatigue, and enhance mood. Tailored exercise programs focusing on strength, flexibility, and cardiovascular health are beneficial.

- **Avoiding Tobacco and Limiting Alcohol**. Refraining from smoking and limiting alcohol consumption can reduce the risk of recurrence and other health issues.

Emotional and Psychological Well-Being

1. Coping with Emotional Changes:

- **Anxiety and Depression**: It is common for survivors to experience anxiety about recurrence and depression due to changes in their life. Professional counseling, support groups, and sometimes medications can help manage these feelings.

- **Identity and Self-Esteem:** The experience of cancer can alter one's sense of identity and self-worth. Engaging in activities that promote self-esteem and finding new passions can aid in this adjustment.

2. Building a Support Network:

- **Family and Friends**: Leaning on close relationships provides emotional support. Open communication about needs and feelings helps strengthen these bonds.

- **Support Groups**: Connecting with other prostate cancer survivors through support groups can provide a sense of community and shared experience.

- **Professional Support**: Psychologists, counselors, and social workers specializing in cancer survivorship can offer professional guidance and support.

Sexual Health and Intimacy
1. Open Communication

- **With Partners:**. Honest conversations about sexual health, expectations, and any changes in sexual function are essential for maintaining intimacy and understanding in relationships.

- **With Healthcare Providers:** Discussing concerns with doctors can lead to appropriate referrals and treatments for sexual health issues.

2. Treatment Options:

- **Medications**: PDE5 inhibitors (such as Viagra) can help manage erectile dysfunction.

- **Therapies**: Penile rehabilitation programs, including vacuum erection devices and penile injections, can improve sexual function.

-**Counseling**: Sex therapy and counseling can help address emotional and psychological aspects of sexual health.

Financial and Practical Considerations

1. **Understanding Insurance and Financial Resources**

   - Navigating insurance coverage and understanding benefits is crucial. Survivors should explore all available resources, including patient assistance programs and financial counseling services.

2. **Managing Employment and Legal Issues:**

   - **Returning to Work**: Transitioning back to work may require adjustments. Discussing accommodations with employers can help ease this transition.

   - **Legal Rights**: Understanding legal rights related to employment and insurance ensures that survivors are protected and supported.

Finding Purpose and Moving Forward
1. Reevaluating Life Goals:

- Personal Growth**: Many survivors find new meaning and purpose after their cancer experience. Engaging in activities that align with personal values and passions can foster personal growth.

- **Community Involvement**: Volunteering, advocacy, and participating in cancer awareness initiatives can provide a sense of purpose and contribute to the greater good.

2. Continual Learning and Adaptation:

- Staying Informed: Keeping up-to-date with the latest research and developments in prostate cancer care helps survivors make informed decisions about their health.

- **Adapting to Change**: Flexibility and adaptability are crucial in navigating the ongoing changes and challenges that may arise during survivorship.

Building a Survivorship Care Plan

1. Creating a Personalized Plan:

- Collaborating with healthcare providers to develop a survivorship care plan tailored to individual needs ensures comprehensive post-treatment care.

2. Components of a Care Plan:

- **Follow-Up Schedule:** Outlining regular check-ups, tests, and screenings.

Management of Side Effects:: Strategies for managing long-term and late effects of treatment.

- **Health Promotion**: Guidelines for diet, exercise, and healthy lifestyle choices.

- **Resources and Support**: Information on support services, financial resources, and community programs.

Survivorship is a journey that encompasses more than just the absence of disease. It involves navigating the physical, emotional, and practical aspects of life after cancer treatment. By understanding the multifaceted nature of survivorship and utilizing the resources and strategies outlined in this chapter, prostate cancer survivors can move forward with confidence, resilience, and a renewed sense of purpose. This phase of the cancer journey is not just about survival but about thriving and living life to its fullest potential.

CHAPTER 11: Prostate Cancer and Sexual Minorities: Special Treatment and Recovery Considerations for Gay and Bisexual Men

Prostate cancer affects men across all demographics, including sexual minorities such as gay and bisexual men. These groups may face unique challenges in terms of treatment, recovery, and emotional support. Understanding and addressing these specific needs is crucial for providing comprehensive and inclusive care. This chapter explores the particular considerations and strategies for managing prostate cancer in gay and bisexual men, ensuring that their treatment and recovery are as effective and supportive as possible.

Understanding Unique Challenges

1. Medical and Social Barriers

- **Healthcare Discrimination**: Gay and bisexual men often face discrimination and bias in healthcare settings, which can affect their willingness to seek timely care and disclose important health information.

- **Lack of Provider Knowledge:** Many healthcare providers may lack specific knowledge about the health needs of sexual minorities, leading to less effective communication and care.

- **Underreporting Symptoms:** Fear of discrimination may cause some men to underreport symptoms, leading to delayed diagnoses and treatments.

2. Sexual Health Considerations

- **Sexual Function and Preferences**: Prostate cancer treatments can significantly impact sexual function, which can be particularly concerning for gay and bisexual men whose sexual practices may rely heavily on prostate health.

- Identity and Relationships: Changes in sexual function can affect self-identity and relationships, potentially leading to psychological distress.

- **Anal Intercourse**: The prostate plays a significant role in sexual pleasure for some men who engage in receptive anal intercourse. Changes to prostate function or the experience of anal pleasure post-treatment are important considerations.

3.Support Systems

- Social Support Gay and bisexual men may have different social support structures, which can influence their emotional well-being and recovery.

- **Community Resources:** Access to LGBTQ+ friendly resources and support groups can be limited, affecting the quality of support received during and after treatment.

- **Family Dynamics**: Family acceptance and support vary widely, impacting emotional and practical support systems.

Special Treatment Considerations

1. Communication with Healthcare Providers

- **Open Dialogue?** Encouraging open and honest communication with healthcare providers about sexual orientation and practices is essential for receiving personalized and effective care.

- **Provider Education** : Patients should feel empowered to educate their providers about their specific needs if the providers lack this knowledge.

- **Disclosure Comfort**: Providers should create a comfortable environment that encourages disclosure of sexual orientation and practices without fear of judgment or discrimination.

2. Treatment Decision-Making:

- Tailored Approaches Treatment plans should be tailored to consider the sexual practices and preferences of gay and bisexual men. For example, certain surgical approaches or radiation techniques might be preferred to minimize impact on sexual function.

- **Impact on Sexual Function**: Understanding the potential impacts of different treatments on sexual function, including erectile function and anal sex, is crucial. Discussing these impacts with a knowledgeable provider can help in making informed decisions.

- **Hormone Therapy** Hormone therapy, commonly used in prostate cancer treatment, can affect libido and sexual function. Discussing these potential side effects and exploring ways to mitigate them is important for maintaining quality of life.

3. Rehabilitation and Recovery:

- **Penile Rehabilitation::** Post-treatment strategies, such as medications (e.g., PDE5 inhibitors), vacuum erection devices, and penile injections, can help in maintaining sexual function.

- **Pelvic Floor Exercises** : These exercises can help in regaining urinary control and improving sexual function post-surgery or radiation.

Emotional and Psychological Well-Being
1. Coping with Emotional Changes

- **Anxiety and Depression**: It is common for survivors to experience anxiety about recurrence and depression due to changes in their life. Professional counseling, support groups, and sometimes medications can help manage these feelings.

- **Identity and Self-Esteem**: The experience of cancer can alter one's sense of identity and self-worth. Engaging in activities that promote self-esteem and finding new passions can aid in this adjustment.

- **Stigma and Isolation**: Gay and bisexual men may face additional stigma related to both their cancer and their sexual orientation, leading to feelings of isolation.

2. Building a Support Network:

- **Family and Friends: Leaning on close relationships provides emotional support. Open communication about needs and feelings helps strengthen these bonds.

- **Connecting** with other prostate cancer survivors through support groups can provide a sense of community and shared experience.

- **Professional Support**: Psychologists, counselors, and social workers specializing in cancer survivorship can offer professional guidance and support.

- **Online Communities**: Online forums and social media groups can offer support and resources, especially if local LGBTQ+ friendly groups are not available.

3. Sexual Health and Intimacy

   - Open Communication:

   - With Partners: Honest conversations about sexual health, expectations, and any changes in sexual function are essential for maintaining intimacy and understanding in relationships.

   - With Healthcare Providers: Discussing concerns with doctors can lead to appropriate referrals and treatments for sexual health issues.

   - Therapy Options:

   - **Medications**,: PDE5 inhibitors (such as Viagra) can help manage erectile dysfunction.

   -**Therapies**: Penile rehabilitation programs, including vacuum erection devices and penile injections, can improve sexual function.

   - **Counseling**: Sex therapy and counseling can help address emotional and psychological aspects of sexual health.

Navigating Healthcare Systems

1. Finding Inclusive Care

- **LGBTQ+ Health Centers**: Seeking care at health centers known for their inclusive practices can improve the quality of care and comfort level of patients.

- **Online Resources:** Utilizing online resources and forums can help in finding LGBTQ+ friendly healthcare providers and support networks.

2. Advocacy and Empowerment

- Patient Advocacy Patients should feel empowered to advocate for their needs and seek second opinions if they are not receiving the care they deserve.

- **Community Involvement:** Engaging with LGBTQ+ advocacy groups can provide additional support and resources.

3. Legal Protections

- **Know Your Rights**l: Understanding legal protections regarding healthcare discrimination can empower patients to stand up for their rights.

- **Patient Confidentiality**: Ensuring that healthcare providers respect and protect patient confidentiality is crucial for building trust and open communication.

Financial and Practical Considerations

1. Understanding Insurance and Financial Resources:

- Navigating insurance coverage and understanding benefits is crucial. Survivors should explore all available resources, including patient assistance programs and financial counseling services.

- **Employment and Legal Issues:**

- Returning to Work Transitioning back to work may require adjustments. Discussing accommodations with employers can help ease this transition.

- **Legal Rights**: Understanding legal rights related to employment and insurance ensures that survivors are protected and supported.

- **Financial Assistance Programs**: Many organizations offer financial assistance for medical bills, medication, and living expenses. It's important to research and utilize these resources.

Enhancing Quality of Life

1. Reevaluating Life Goals:

- **Personal Growth**: Many survivors find new meaning and purpose after their cancer experience. Engaging in activities that align with personal values and passions can foster personal growth.

-        **Community   Involvement**: Volunteering, advocacy, and participating in cancer awareness initiatives can provide a sense of purpose and contribute to the greater good.

2. Continual Learning and Adaptation

- Staying Informed: Keeping up-to-date with the latest research and developments in prostate cancer care helps survivors make informed decisions about their health.

- **Adapting to Change:** Flexibility and adaptability are crucial in navigating the ongoing changes and challenges that may arise during survivorship.

3. Building a Survivorship Care Plan:

- Creating a Personalized Plan Collaborating with healthcare providers to develop a survivorship care plan tailored to individual needs ensures comprehensive post-treatment care.

- **Components of a Care Plan**:

- **Follow-Up Schedule**: Outlining regular check-ups, tests, and screenings.

- **Management of Side Effects**: Strategies for managing long-term and late effects of treatment.

- **Health Promotion**: Guidelines for diet, exercise, and healthy lifestyle choices.

- Resources and Support: Information on support services, financial resources, and community programs

Gay and bisexual men with prostate cancer face unique challenges that require special consideration in treatment and recovery. By fostering open communication with healthcare providers, tailoring treatment plans to individual needs, and accessing supportive resources, these patients can achieve better outcomes and maintain a higher quality of life. This chapter highlights the importance of understanding and addressing the specific needs of sexual minorities, ensuring that prostate cancer care is inclusive, comprehensive, and compassionate. Through informed decision-making, emotional support, and community involvement, gay and bisexual men can navigate their cancer journey with resilience and hope.

CHAPTER 12: Addressing Erectile Dysfunction Post-Treatment of Prostate Cancer

Erectile dysfunction (ED) is a common and often distressing side effect of prostate cancer treatments. The prostate gland plays a crucial role in male sexual function, and treatments such as surgery, radiation, and hormone therapy can impact the nerves, blood vessels, and tissues involved in achieving and maintaining an erection. Understanding the causes, preventive measures, and treatment options for ED is vital for men undergoing prostate cancer treatment to maintain their quality of life and intimate relationships.

Understanding Erectile Dysfunction in Prostate Cancer Survivors

1. Causes of Erectile Dysfunction Post-Treatment:

\- **Surgical Treatment (Radical Prostatectomy)**

\- **Nerve Damage:** The nerves responsible for erections run close to the prostate gland. During radical prostatectomy, these nerves can be damaged or severed, leading to ED.

- **Vascular Damage**: Surgery can also affect the blood vessels that supply the penis, compromising blood flow and erectile function.

- **Radiation Therapy**

- **Nerve and Tissue Damage**: Radiation can cause fibrosis (scarring) and damage to the erectile tissues and nerves.

- **Delayed Onset**:: ED related to radiation therapy may develop gradually over months or years.

- **Hormone Therapy (Androgen Deprivation Therapy, ADT):**

- **Hormonal Changes**: Lowering testosterone levels can significantly decrease libido and impair erectile function. Testosterone is crucial for maintaining erectile health.

Addressing Erectile Dysfunction: Preventive Measures and Early Interventions

1. Pre-Treatment Counseling and Baseline Assessment:

- **Education and Expectation Setting:** Discuss potential side effects of prostate cancer treatments with patients before starting therapy. Understanding the risk of ED and available interventions can help manage expectations.

- **Baseline Erectile Function::** Assess erectile function before treatment to tailor post-treatment strategies effectively.

2. Nerve-Sparing Surgical Techniques:

- **Nerve-Sparing Radical Prostatectomy:** Surgeons can use techniques to preserve the neurovascular bundles that control erections. The success of this approach depends on the tumor's location and extent.

3. Early Rehabilitation Strategies:

- **Penile Rehabilitation Programs:** Early intervention with penile rehabilitation can help preserve erectile function. This may include the use of medications, devices, and exercises to maintain penile health and prevent tissue damage.

Treatment Options for Erectile Dysfunction

1. Phosphodiesterase Type 5 Inhibitors (PDE5 Inhibitors):

- **Common Medications**: Sildenafil (Viagra), Tadalafil (Cialis), Vardenafil (Levitra), and Avanafil (Stendra).

- **Mechanism of Action:** These drugs enhance the effects of nitric oxide, a natural chemical the body produces to relax penile muscles. This increases blood flow and allows an erection in response to sexual stimulation.

- **Usage and Effectiveness**: PDE5 inhibitors are often the first line of treatment. They are taken orally before sexual activity and have varying onset times and durations of action. Effectiveness depends on the extent of nerve damage.

2. Intracavernosal Injections (ICI):

-**Medications Used**: Alprostadil, Papaverine, Phentolamine.

- **Mechanism of Action**: These drugs are injected directly into the penile tissue, causing an erection by expanding blood vessels and increasing blood flow.

- **Usage:** Patients are trained to self-administer injections. Erections typically occur within 5 to 20 minutes and last about an hour.

3. Vacuum Erection Devices (VED):

- **How They Work:** VEDs create a vacuum around the penis, drawing blood into the erectile tissue. A constriction ring is then applied to maintain the erection.

- **Usage**: This mechanical approach is non-invasive and can be effective for men who cannot use or do not respond to medications.

4. Intraurethral Therapy:

- **Medicated Urethral System for Erections (MUSE):** Alprostadil suppositories are inserted into the urethra using a special applicator.

- **Mechanism of Action:** Alprostadil promotes blood flow to the penis, inducing an erection.

- **Usage**: The method is less invasive than injections but can be less effective for some men.

5. Penile Implants:

- Types of Implants:

- **Inflatable Implants**: Consist of cylinders implanted in the penis, a pump in the scrotum, and a reservoir in the abdomen. The pump transfers fluid into the cylinders to create an erection.

- **Malleable Implants**: Consist of bendable rods implanted in the penis, which can be manually adjusted to an erect position.

- **Usage and Considerations**: Penile implants are considered when other treatments fail. They provide a permanent solution for ED but require surgical implantation.

6. Lifestyle Modifications and Natural Remedies:

- **Healthy Diet**: A diet rich in fruits, vegetables, whole grains, and lean proteins supports vascular health and erectile function.

- **Regular Exercise**: Physical activity improves cardiovascular health and blood flow, aiding erectile function.

- **Weight Management**: Maintaining a healthy weight reduces the risk of ED.

- **Stress Reduction:** Stress and anxiety can worsen ED. Techniques such as mindfulness, meditation, and therapy can help manage stress.

- **Avoiding Tobacco and Limiting Alcohol:** Smoking and excessive alcohol intake can impair blood flow and nerve function, exacerbating ED.

Psychological and Emotional Support

1. Impact of ED on Mental Health::

- **Depression and Anxiety:** ED can lead to feelings of inadequacy, depression, and anxiety, affecting overall mental health and quality of life.

- **Relationship Strain**: ED can strain intimate relationships, leading to communication issues and decreased satisfaction.

2. Counseling and Therapy:

- **Sex Therapy**: Working with a sex therapist can help address the psychological aspects of ED, improve communication with partners, and develop coping strategies.

- **Couples Therapy**: Therapy for both partners can enhance mutual understanding, support, and intimacy.

3. Support Groups:

- **Peer Support:** Joining support groups for prostate cancer survivors can provide emotional support, share experiences, and reduce feelings of isolation.

-**Online Communities:** Online forums and social media groups offer a platform for sharing information, advice, and encouragement.

Addressing erectile dysfunction post-treatment of prostate cancer is a multifaceted challenge that requires a comprehensive approach. From preventive measures and early interventions to various treatment options and psychological support, managing ED is crucial for maintaining quality of life and intimate relationships. Open communication with healthcare providers, personalized treatment plans, and access to supportive resources are essential for navigating this aspect of prostate cancer survivorship. By understanding and addressing the complexities of ED, prostate cancer survivors can achieve better outcomes and improve their overall well-being.

CHAPTER 13: Confronting Metastatic Cancer: Therapeutic Strategies

Metastatic prostate cancer, also known as advanced or stage IV prostate cancer, occurs when cancer has spread beyond the prostate gland to other parts of the body, such as bones, lymph nodes, or other organs. Confronting metastatic cancer requires a multifaceted approach that combines various therapeutic strategies to manage the disease, alleviate symptoms, and improve quality of life. This chapter delves into the comprehensive therapeutic strategies for managing metastatic prostate cancer.

Understanding Metastatic Prostate Cancer

Prostate cancer metastasis typically follows a predictable pattern, first spreading to nearby tissues and lymph nodes, then to bones, and eventually to other organs. The most common sites of metastasis for prostate cancer are:

1. Bones: Often the first site of metastasis, leading to pain, fractures, and other skeletal-related events.

2. Lymph Nodes: Cancer can spread to pelvic and retroperitoneal lymph nodes.

3. Organs: Less commonly, prostate cancer can spread to the liver, lungs, and other organs.

Therapeutic Strategies for Metastatic Prostate Cancer

The management of metastatic prostate cancer involves systemic therapies that target cancer cells throughout the body, local therapies to control symptoms and complications, and supportive care to improve overall quality of life.

1. Androgen Deprivation Therapy (ADT)

As discussed in the previous chapter, ADT is the primary systemic therapy for metastatic prostate cancer. It aims to reduce the levels of androgens (male hormones) that fuel cancer growth.

Mechanisms of ADT:

- **LHRH Agonists and Antagonists**: Reduce testosterone production.

- **Anti-Androgens**: Block the action of androgens.

- **Androgen Synthesis Inhibitors**: Inhibit androgen production.ADT is often the first line of treatment for metastatic prostate cancer and can be combined with other therapies to enhance effectiveness.

2. Chemotherapy

Chemotherapy uses drugs to kill rapidly dividing cancer cells. It is particularly useful when prostate cancer becomes resistant to hormonal therapy (castration-resistant prostate cancer, CRPC).

Common Chemotherapy Agents

-**Docetaxel:** A taxane-based chemotherapy that disrupts microtubule function, essential for cell division.

- **Cabazitaxel**: Another taxane effective in patients who have progressed after docetaxel treatment.

Benefits:

- Reduces tumor burden.

- Alleviates symptoms such as pain.

- Prolongs survival in metastatic castration-resistant prostate cancer (mCRPC).

3. Novel Hormonal Agents

Recent advancements have led to the development of new hormonal therapies that offer benefits beyond traditional ADT.

Examples

- **Abiraterone Acetate (Zytiga):** Inhibits CYP17, a key enzyme in androgen biosynthesis.

- **Enzalutamide (Xtandi):** An androgen receptor inhibitor that blocks multiple steps in the androgen receptor signaling pathway.

- **Apalutamide (Erleada) and Darolutamide (Nubeqa):** Newer androgen receptor inhibitors with fewer side effects.

These agents are used in combination with ADT for enhanced efficacy, particularly in mCRPC.

4. Immunotherapy

Immunotherapy harnesses the body's immune system to target and destroy cancer cells. In prostate cancer, the most notable immunotherapy is sipuleucel-T (Provenge).

Sipuleucel-T (Provenge):

- Mechanism: A personalized vaccine made from the patient's own immune cells, designed to stimulate an immune response against prostate cancer cells.

- **Benefits**: Can extend survival in certain patients with asymptomatic or minimally symptomatic mCRPC.

5. Targeted Therapy

Targeted therapies are designed to specifically target molecular pathways essential for cancer cell survival and proliferation.

PARP Inhibitors:

- **Olaparib (Lynparza) and Rucaparib (Rubraca):** Used in patients with mutations in DNA repair genes (e.g., BRCA1/2).
- **Mechanism**: Inhibit PARP enzymes, which are involved in DNA repair, leading to cancer cell death in tumors with defective DNA repair mechanisms.

6. Radionuclide Therapy

Radionuclide therapy involves the use of radioactive substances to target cancer cells.

Radium-223 Dichloride (Xofigo):
- **Mechanism**: Mimics calcium and targets bone metastases, delivering localized radiation.
- **Benefits**: Reduces bone pain, decreases skeletal-related events, and prolongs

survival in patients with bone-dominant mCRPC.

7. Bone-Targeted Therapies

Given the high propensity of prostate cancer to metastasize to bones, bone-targeted therapies are crucial.

Bisphosphonates:
- **Zoledronic Acid (Zometa):** Inhibits bone resorption, reduces bone pain, and prevents skeletal-related events.

RANK Ligand Inhibitors:
- **Denosumab (Xgeva):** Prevents bone loss by inhibiting the RANK ligand pathway, reducing the risk of fractures and other skeletal complications.

8. Radiation Therapy

Radiation therapy can be used to control symptoms and manage localized areas of metastasis.

External Beam Radiation Therapy (EBRT):

- **Use**: Targets specific bone metastases to alleviate pain and prevent fractures.

- **Benefits**: Provides symptomatic relief and improves quality of life.

9. Multimodal Approaches

Combining multiple therapeutic strategies can offer better control of metastatic prostate cancer and improve patient outcomes.

Examples:

- **ADT + Chemotherapy:** Combining ADT with docetaxel has shown improved survival in patients with newly diagnosed metastatic hormone-sensitive prostate cancer.

- **ADT + Novel Hormonal Agents**: Using abiraterone or enzalutamide with ADT provides better disease control compared to ADT alone.

- **Immunotherapy + Radiation:** Combining sipuleucel-T with radiation to enhance the immune response against cancer cells.

10. Supportive Care

Supportive care is integral to managing the symptoms and side effects associated with metastatic prostate cancer and its treatments.

Pain Management:

- Medications: NSAIDs, opioids, and bisphosphonates for bone pain.

- Radiation Therapy: For localized pain control.

Nutritional Support

- **Dietary Interventions**: Tailored to manage weight loss, maintain strength, and support overall health.

Psychosocial Support:

- **Counseling and Support Groups**: Address emotional and psychological challenges.

- **Palliative Care::** Focuses on improving quality of life through symptom management and holistic support.

Confronting metastatic prostate cancer involves a comprehensive and multidisciplinary approach that integrates various therapeutic strategies. From hormonal therapy and chemotherapy to novel targeted treatments and supportive care, the goal is to manage the disease effectively, alleviate symptoms, and improve the patient's quality of life. With ongoing research and advancements in treatment options, the outlook for patients with metastatic prostate cancer continues to improve, offering hope for better outcomes and prolonged survival.

CONCLUSION: A Journey of Hope and Healing

Prostate cancer, often surrounded by fear and uncertainty, demands a comprehensive approach to understanding, managing, and overcoming the disease. Throughout this book, we have journeyed through the intricate landscape of prostate cancer, from its biological underpinnings to the various strategies employed in its detection, treatment, and ongoing management. As we conclude, it is essential to reflect on the key lessons and insights that underscore this journey of hope and healing.

Understanding and Awareness

Knowledge is the foundation of empowerment in the fight against prostate cancer. Understanding the anatomy and physiology of the prostate, recognizing the risk factors, and being aware of the symptoms are crucial steps in early detection and effective treatment. Regular screenings, such as PSA tests and digital rectal exams, play a pivotal role in identifying the disease in its early stages, when it is most treatable.

Prevention and Lifestyle Choices

While some risk factors, like genetics and age, are beyond our control, lifestyle choices can significantly impact prostate health. Adopting a balanced diet rich in fruits, vegetables, and whole grains, coupled with regular exercise, can contribute to overall well-being and potentially reduce the risk of prostate cancer. Limiting alcohol consumption and avoiding smoking are also essential preventive measures that support not only prostate health but general health.

Advancements in Treatment

The landscape of prostate cancer treatment has evolved remarkably, offering patients a range of options tailored to their specific needs. From surgical interventions like radical prostatectomy to innovative therapies such as immunotherapy and targeted treatments, the arsenal against prostate cancer is more robust than ever. Hormonal therapy and radiation therapy continue to be mainstays in managing advanced stages of the disease, while emerging therapies and clinical trials offer hope for the future.

Personalized Care and Survivorship

Prostate cancer treatment is not a one-size-fits-all approach. Personalizing care based on the unique characteristics of each patient's cancer and their overall health is critical. This includes considering factors such as the stage of cancer, the patient's age, and any underlying health conditions. Survivorship care plans, which focus on monitoring, managing long-term side effects, and maintaining a healthy lifestyle, are essential for improving the quality of life for survivors.

Emotional and Psychosocial Support

The emotional and psychological impact of prostate cancer cannot be overstated. From the initial diagnosis through treatment and beyond, patients and their families face significant challenges. Access to counseling, support groups, and mental health services is vital in providing the necessary emotional support. Open communication with healthcare providers and loved ones can also alleviate anxiety and foster a supportive environment.

The Importance of Research and Advocacy

Continued research is paramount in advancing our understanding of prostate cancer and developing new treatments. Clinical trials and studies contribute to the growing body of knowledge, leading to breakthroughs that improve patient outcomes. Advocacy for increased funding, awareness campaigns, and education efforts are essential in supporting research initiatives and ensuring that patients have access to the best possible care.

A Message of Hope

Despite the challenges posed by prostate cancer, there is a profound message of hope embedded in the advances in medical science, the resilience of patients, and the support of families and communities. Survivors of prostate cancer exemplify strength and perseverance, and their stories inspire others facing similar battles.

As we conclude this book, it is our hope that the information, insights, and personal stories shared within these pages have provided you with a comprehensive understanding of prostate cancer and the tools to navigate your own journey or support a loved one. Whether you are a patient, caregiver, or healthcare provider, remember that you are not alone. There is a vast network of resources, support systems, and advancements in medical science that can guide you through this journey.

Together, we can confront prostate cancer with knowledge, compassion, and unwavering hope. By staying informed, making healthy choices, and seeking the best possible care, we can transform the experience of prostate cancer from one of fear and uncertainty to one of empowerment and healing.